# Neuro-Mass

## The Ultimate System
## for Spectacular Strength

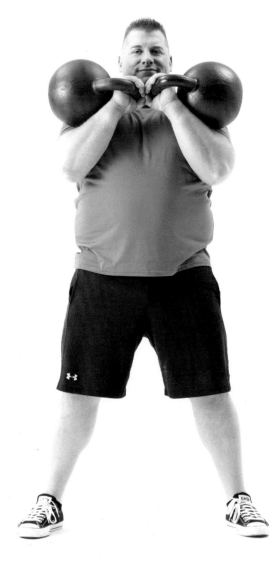

## By Jon Bruney

# Neuro-Mass

## The Ultimate System for Spectacular Strength

### By Jon Bruney

A Dragon Door Publications, Inc. production
All rights under International and Pan-American Copyright conventions.
Published in the United States by: Dragon Door Publications, Inc.
5 East County Rd B, #3 • Little Canada, MN 55117
Tel: (651) 487-2180 • Fax: (651) 487-3954
Credit card orders: 1-800-899-5111 • Email: support@dragondoor.com • Website: www.dragondoor.com

ISBN 10: 0-938045-99-7    ISBN 13: 978-0-938045-99-1
This edition first published in September, 2013
Printed in China

Book design and cover by Derek Brigham • www.dbrigham.com • bigd@dbrigham.com
Photography by Don Pitlik

DISCLAIMER: The author and publisher of this material are not responsible in any manner whatsoever for any injury that may occur through following the instructions contained in this material. The activities, physical and otherwise, described herein for informational purposes only, may be too strenuous or dangerous for some people and the reader(s) should consult a physician before engaging in them.

# TABLE OF CONTENTS

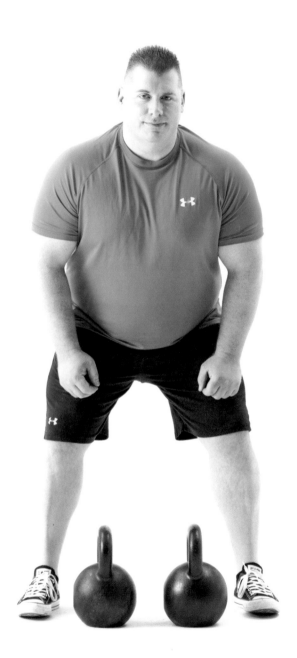

# Acknowledgements

To my Lord and Savior Jesus Christ

To my Wife Amy and Daughters JoLynn and Jonna

To my Mother, Father, and brothers who have
always been my biggest cheerleaders

To the Pressing The Limits Team

To the people of Zion Missionary Church-
Thanks for partnering with me

To John Brookfield who gave me my start in the
world of Strongman

To Mike Gillette- Thanks for the encouragement

To John Du Cane for making this project possible

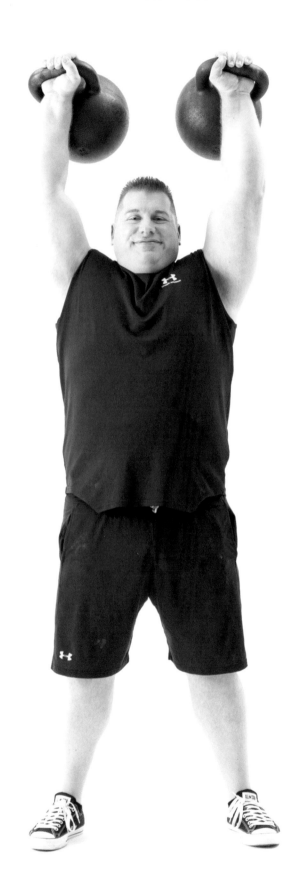

# FOREWORD

# A new approach to an old vexing problem

## by Marty Gallagher

Jon Bruney is a very large, very fit performing strongman. Jon is a thinking man who has developed his own very unique approach towards answering the eternal dilemma of the hardcore athlete: what protocols and procedures work best for morphing human performance from mundane into sublime, while concurrently and simultaneously morphing the human physique from ordinary into extraordinary?

Big Jon, whom I have never met, has a protégé-mentor relationship with grip grand maestro John Brookfield. Big Jon is a longtime performing strongman and coming from this unique blended background, one sees how Bruney's experiences would certainly bend and shape his philosophy towards all things power, strength and muscle-related. Aristotle once said, "We *are* what we do repeatedly."

I am somewhat familiar with the grueling training regimen Brookfield champions. I hope I am doing him justice when I say that for me, Brookfield's approach is a lot more than that of a grip master. Brookfield, Bruney, Steve Justa and other iron pioneers champion what I would call "strength/endurance" or "sustained strength." To excel in the sustained strength world a man needs a high tolerance for pain—pain is factually too strong a word. Pain should be reserved for injurious happenings and occurrences; what we are talking about is major league, self-inflicted physical *discomfort*.

Pain tolerance can be increased over time. Increasing the ability to tolerate pain requires a purposeful visiting and revisiting of current tolerance limits. Over time we push back existing boundaries and limits. The ability to withstand a certain amount of intense physical discomfort is a mighty attribute for any real man (or woman) to possess. Arnold Schwarzenegger once noted, "Those that can stand deep and repeated trips into the pain zone might become a champion—those that cannot have no chance of ever excelling."

It is purely conjecture on my part, but one can easily imagine how grueling grip training would steel the mind for the intense protocols Jon Bruney offers up. Grip mastery is as much mental as physical; grip work requires long, excruciating isometric holds clutching ponderous poundage for protracted periods. High level grip work is about steeling the mind to ignore the very real, very unpleasant burning sensations in the working muscles. The idea of isometrics is very big in both Jon and John's approach. This is a fantastic thing because isometrics is a legitimate exercise mode worthy of resurrection.

I remember reading one memorable Brookfield article in *MILO* that involved driving to the country (in my case I already live there) and knocking on a farmer's door to obtain permission—no, not to date his gorgeous daughter—but instead to ask if he could push with all his might against a giant, immovable, one-ton hay bale that lay in that farmer's field. I often drive by monster bales in my rural neighborhood and wonder what my reaction would be were I to be driving by and suddenly came upon giant men screaming, frothing at the mouths like mentally insane people; grunting, swearing, pushing with their might against seemingly immovable objects.

Any human over age 6 could grok the "impossibility" of moving the giant bale and would avoid such taxing, seemingly mindless activity. Little do civilians understand that Brookfield was looking for an isometric/isotonic workout of the first magnitude; hay bale isometrics was madness rooted in logic. That Brookfield succeeded in pushing the one-ton bale clear across the field is beside the point. The logic behind the madness was a method, a protocol, a strategy for increasing *sustained strength* by engaging in protracted isometric and isotonic struggle. Brookfield tilts at hay bales like Don Quixote tilted at windmills.

Out of this tradition of grip and pain tolerance and isometrics and strongman competition sprang Bruney. Strongman feats are all about sustained strength: drag giant chains, carry heavy weights for distance, pick up multiple stones—strength alone, pure strength, one rep max strength, will not win you a strongman competition. Strongman in its current state should not be called 'World's Strongest Man' that title should go to the one-rep max champ—the appropriate title would be "World's Strongest Strength/Endurance Athlete."

So how does one go about attaining sustained strength and all the fabulous attributes that accompany its acquisition? Jon Bruney offers us his solution in this book. The premise of this book is to provide the reader with a new and "revolutionary" system that provides the diligent user both absolute strength and sustained strength along with maximum muscle hypertrophy, all by using a unique protocol that couples different strength methodologies.

The guts of this book, to my way of thinking, is Jon's three-part "set" that maximally taxes a multitude of pathways. Bruney's approach creates maximum muscular exhaustion or muscle "inroad," as we used to say in the 1980s. Maximal inroad occurs when a muscle, or group of muscles, is totally devastated on a variety of levels. Jon has devised a devilishly exhausting protocol that consists of three parts: grind, explode, and iso-push. Target muscle or muscle groups are routinely shattered, inducing muscle hypertrophy, assuming you don't wuss out on the poundage. Jon's procedure makes terrific sense….

• *Grinds:* slow, controlled exercises that require maximum body tension. Grinds make light weights heavy and ingrain proper technique. We start with grinds.

• *Dynamic Power Drills:* explosive movements require power and speed. The purposeful use of momentum delivers enhanced effect.

• *Isometrics:* push or pull against an immovable object. The joint-angle and muscle-length remain constant for the duration of the isometric contraction.

Jon features a telling quote by Mike Mentzer, "Anything that you can do to make your workout harder is a step in the right direction." Jon has definitely picked up Mike's battle flag and added a few Brookfield-ian influenced intensity amplifiers along the way.

The Bruney Neuro-Set is pure conjured-up hell: you commence the set by grinding the poundage, purposefully slowing the rep speed on both ascent and descent. After a predetermined number of grind reps, commence performing high velocity ballistic reps making use of speed and momentum. Finish this man-breaker set with a final push-or-pull-your-guts-out isometric finale that targets the muscle(s) already shattered in the grind/explosive portion of the set. Ouch! This has got to hurt! Sissies need not apply.

Anyone looking to blast themselves out of whatever quagmire they find themselves mired in need look no further than the protocols and strategies outlined in this excellent book. Any team sport athlete would be well advised to immediately commence a cycle incorporating Jon Bruney's methods. Athletes need what Jon is offering: pure power combined with amazing capacity for sustained and continual strength output. This type of training can provide users an entirely new strength approach that will prove particularly beneficial to fighters, athletes, military and law enforcement types. The approach will also allow regular folks a method with which to round out their current capacities and capabilities.

Let us not always and continually play to our strengths, let us identify, embrace and celebrate our physical weaknesses. As all real pros know, working weak points is where the real gains lie. Bruney's book mercilessly attacks weak points and this is always a recipe for tangible progress.

Marty Gallagher
May 2013

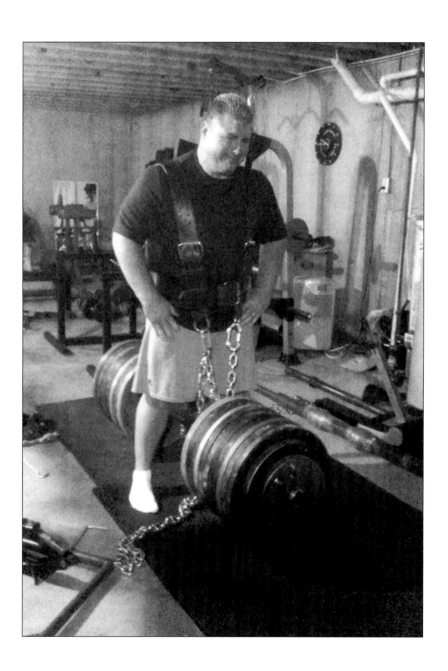

# INTRODUCTION

*"Unless we change our direction, we are
likely to end up where we are headed."*
—Chinese Proverb

**W**hen it comes to physique development, there are many paths one can take. Success or failure in the quest for muscle mass is dependent on choosing the right path. That is why I developed this program. Neuro-Mass provides the fastest means for adding slabs of **functional** muscle to your frame. That's right, *functional* muscle... SMART muscle. Smart muscle is muscle that can multi-task. Neuro-Mass will not only increase your frame, but also turbo-charge your strength and athleticism.

Everyone wants to add muscle, but we all know that it's no easy task. Confusion and misinformation abounds as to how exactly this is accomplished. Neuro-Mass removes the confusion by giving you the **exact protocols** to create an impressive athletic physique. The Neuro-Mass system combines the best kettlebell resistance exercises with a new cutting edge training method called "Neuro-Sets". And these Neuro-Sets create RAPID physique transformation. While most training programs only focus on one approach to create growth, Neuro-Mass uses multiple stressors to create a BIGGER and BETTER body.

Neuro-Mass makes the body smarter by:

- Teaching the nervous system to recruit more muscle fibers.
- Teaching the body to adapt to multiple forms of resistance.
- Teaching the body to bypass genetic performance roadblocks.

Before I share the Neuro-Mass system with you, let me share a little background on myself. I am a world record-holding strongman, trainer, coach, motivational speaker, author, and pastor. My work with competitive athletes includes Olympians and NFL players. Preparing myself, as well as others, for maximum athletic performance has given me insight on how to reach the body's true potential. Out of this experience comes Neuro-Mass.

For those who would join in the pursuit of mass and athleticism…

Welcome to NEURO-MASS

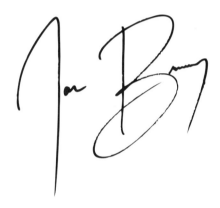

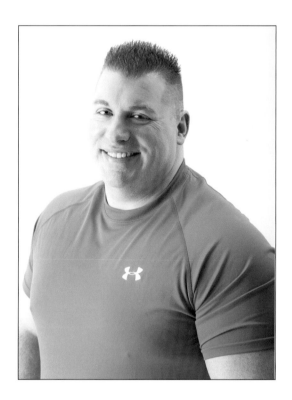

# The Grind-and-Go Principle—The Secret to Athletic Dominance

For the human body to keep its balance while standing still, it requires about 300 muscles to work together. Imagine how much more neuromuscular skill is needed to accomplish feats of athleticism. To achieve elite athletic performance, one must master the ability to change the exertion of muscular force rapidly. I have had many discussions on this topic with my mentor, legendary strongman John Brookfield. We coined the phrase the "grind-and-go principle", as a way to describe this skill.

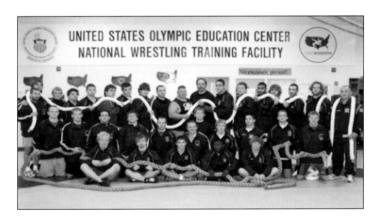

Take for instance, a Greco-Roman wrestling match. I have personally witnessed these elite wrestlers display this skill masterfully. The wrestler will usually start the match by tying up his opponent. There is a "grinding" muscular force being exerted in this position. Then at the opportune time, he throws his opponent to the mat. This represents the "go" or explosive muscular force. Now on the mat, the wrestler will use grinding force to try to turn his opponent's shoulders to the mat for a fall. A wrestler who switches seamlessly from various body locks to throws and suplexes is a perfect example of the grind-and-go principle in action.

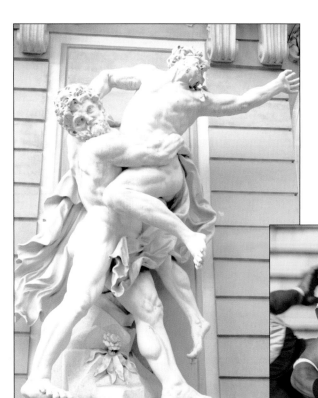

This skill is critical in contact sports such as football. An offensive lineman must explode off the ball into the defender. As impact occurs with the opponent, the lineman must now exert grinding muscular tension to try and control the defender. The player then must be able to release his block, and explode down field to block another defender.

I learned the importance of this skill firsthand when setting world records in truck-pulling. On multiple occasions, John Brookfield and I have pulled large semi-trucks. The pulls were not only feats of strength but also of endurance, as we pulled the trucks for a distance of one mile. To begin the pull, I had to exert maximum grinding tension. I then had to transition to dynamic power to keep the truck moving.

Developing the ability to grind-and-go is the secret to athletic dominance. We all like to win…whether it's setting a lifting PR in the garage, or scoring on the gridiron. It has been said that the only person who likes to lose is probably playing golf with his boss. This is why Neuro-Mass is so important. It is the ONLY training system that delivers the ability to grind and go.

So how exactly does this get accomplished? Enter the Neuro-Set.

# Unleash the POWER of NEURO-SETS

**O**ver the years there have been many different types of training protocols. In the quest for mass and strength we have seen pre-exhaust sets, negatives, x-reps, speed sets, partials, volume training, and so many others. Regardless of method, the goal of all of these protocols is to stimulate growth through maximum muscle recruitment and resistance overload. And over the years, all of these techniques have had their place. But the time has come for a different kind of mass training. A different kind of strength training. It's time for something REVOLUTIONARY. Enter the Neuro-Set...

A Neuro-Set is comprised of three distinct types of exercises all combined into one brutally effective set. The synergistic result of this exercise combination is increased neuro-muscular efficiency and MAXIMUM muscular hypertrophy. This means that the Neuro-Set not only increases muscle size, but also strength and athleticism.

The three types of exercise that make up the Neuro-Set are as follows:

**Grinds** - Slow, controlled exercises that place resistance on large muscle groups. These exercises require total-body tension.

**Dynamic Power Drills** - Performed quickly, these are movements that require power *and* speed. They are ballistic in the concentric portion of the movement and also use momentum to deliver an enhanced eccentric-loading effect.

**Isometrics** - This category of exercise is performed while maintaining a static position. The joint-angle and muscle-length remain constant for the duration of the contraction.

Each one of these exercise types has historically been quite effective on its own. But when they are synergistically combined into a Neuro-Set, they become a powerful force that smashes through the roadblocks of physique transformation. It is like comparing a firecracker with a stick of dynamite.

# The Importance of Grinds:

Kettlebell and bodyweight grinds include squats, pulls, and presses all done in a slow controlled manner. The proper execution of these exercises requires sustained total-body tension. The stress that grinds place on the muscular system leads to hypertrophy. To complete a grind, stabilizer muscles must come into play. This builds tremendous overall structural strength. And when done properly, using the correct rep sequence, grinds have the potential to elicit a productive hormonal response.

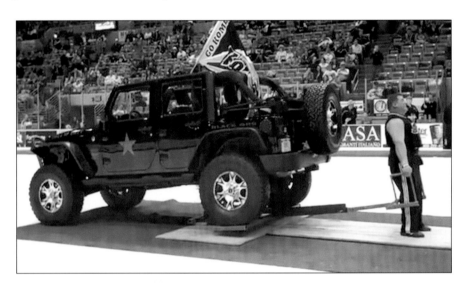

I have used kettlebell grinds to prepare my body for big performance lifts such as deadlifting the back of an SUV. Kettlebell front squats and deadlifts help me to practice generating the tension needed for these massive lifts. They also help by improving my performance groove.

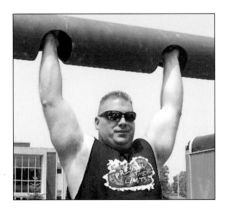

Kettlebell grinds will also point out any weak links in your muscular chain. These exercises teach body proper alignment and output for maximum strength.

Bodyweight grinds, such as the handstand pushup, train my body to press heavy steel strongman logs overhead. Grinds also teach the body to work together as a unit. These exercises increase body control and coordination, which leads to better athletic performance.

# The Importance of Dynamic Power Drills:

These ballistic exercises require explosive acceleration and speed. When using kettlebells for these drills, you create a perpetual deceleration and reloading effect, which increases your ability to generate power. And the extreme deceleration from these exercises develops your body's ability to absorb shock. The explosive drills in Neuro-Mass recruit your fast-twitch muscle fibers, which leads to muscle growth or hypertrophy. The intensity of these drills is such that it leads to a huge increase in your metabolic rate and produces a hybrid effect by enhancing both strength *and* conditioning.

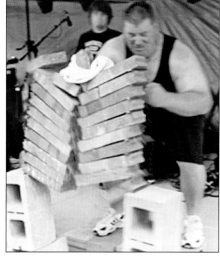

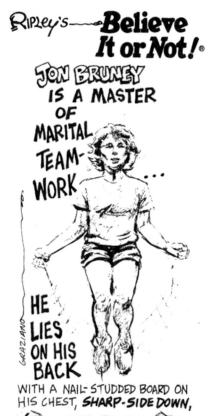

Ripley's— **Believe It or Not!**®

JON BRUNEY IS A MASTER OF MARITAL TEAM-WORK ...

HE LIES ON HIS BACK WITH A NAIL-STUDDED BOARD ON HIS CHEST, *SHARP-SIDE DOWN,* WHILE HIS WIFE AMY JUMPS ROPE ON TOP OF IT!

2-8  © 2005 Ripley Entertainment Inc.

Dynamic power drills are essential to my personal training. These drills prepare my body for incredible breaking feats. I regularly crush slabs of concrete using my fist, a task that requires incredible speed. For the concrete to break, my fist must be able to deliver maximum impact. This type of breaking is the ultimate expression of acceleration and deceleration; the acceleration toward the concrete, followed by the forced deceleration upon impact. I rely on ballistic kettlebell drills to keep me injury-free while performing this kind of feat. And I have seen an increase in my breaking skills as a direct result of this ballistic kettlebell work.

I have used bodyweight dynamic power drills such as the plyometric push-up to prepare for strongman feats that involve absorbing maximum force. One such feat is where I lay under a bed of nails while my wife jumps rope on top of it. Another feat involves dropping a 16 pound bowling ball off a seven foot ladder onto my stomach. Without the ability to absorb impact, I wouldn't survive. Bodyweight dynamic power drills are a great tool for increasing not only explosive power, but also resiliency.

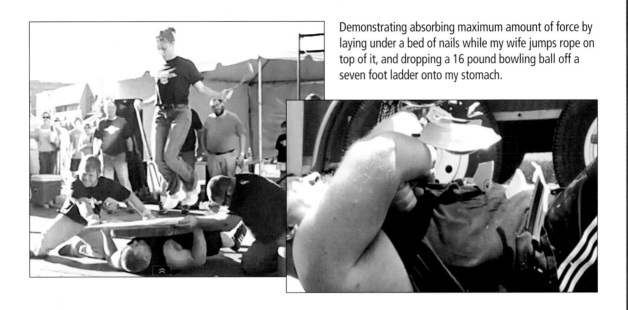

Demonstrating absorbing maximum amount of force by laying under a bed of nails while my wife jumps rope on top of it, and dropping a 16 pound bowling ball off a seven foot ladder onto my stomach.

# The Importance of Isometrics:

Traditional strength training allows the muscles to contract concentrically {while the muscle shortens}, as well as eccentrically {while the muscle lengthens}. Isometric exercise focuses on contracting a muscle *without* changing its length. Imagine pulling a large tent stake that is stuck in the ground. If the stake does not move, this pulling action becomes an isometric exercise. Isometric drills focus on trying to move the unmovable. These exercises have been used for centuries as a way to build unbelievable strength.

Many legendary strongmen have successfully incorporated isometrics into their training regimens. A notable example was the amazing Alexander Zass. Zass was known for his ability to break chains and bend bars. But his most remarkable feats of strength also included:

- Carrying a horse around his shoulders.
- Catching a woman fired from a cannon.
- Walking with a piano strapped to his back.
- Lifting a 500 pound girder with his teeth.
- Being able to absorb punches to his abdomen.

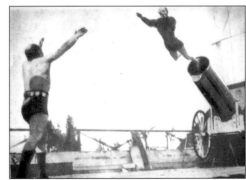

So how did Zass build his amazing strength? Simple. Zass himself credited his extensive use of isometrics. While he was a prisoner of war he performed isometric pulls on his chains and prison bars.

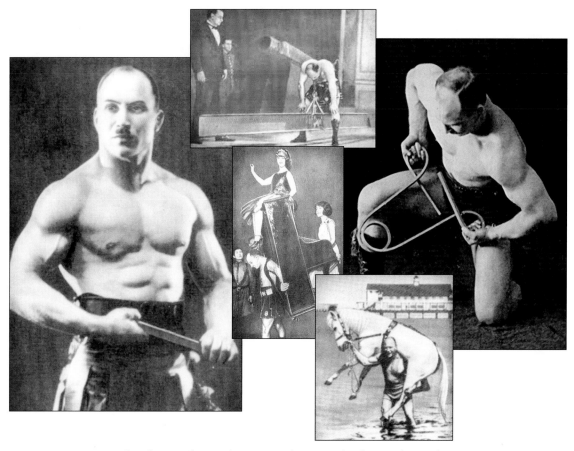

Isometrics can also be performed using only your bodyweight. These are intense contractions resulting from you tensing the muscles and tendons in a flexed position. Many great strongmen have used this technique including Mike Dayton who won Mr. America two times. His feats included breaking police handcuffs, snapping baseball bats in two, and even bending quarters.

Among the feats in my own strength repertoire, my favorite one to perform is called the Human Link. This involves having two Harley Davidson motorcycles attached to my arms. The feat requires me to resist the motorcycles as they attempt to take off in opposite directions, essentially trying to pull me in two. While the feat is extraordinarily difficult to perform, the method I employ to do it is quite simple. I perform an isometric contraction against the resistance of the two motorcycles. And without my extensive background in isometric training, this feat would be impossible to accomplish.

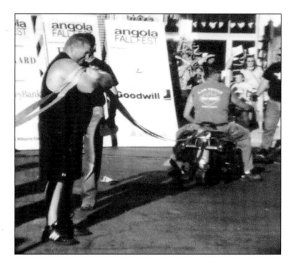

Now let's look at how these three types of exercises are incorporated into the Neuro-Set. For chest and upper body development a **<u>kettlebell Neuro-Set could look like this</u>**:

**GRIND** - Kettlebell bench press
    Immediately followed by:

**DYNAMIC POWER DRILL** - Kettlebell rolling speed press
    Immediately followed by:

**ISOMETRIC** - Kettlebell chest crush.


**<u>A bodyweight Neuro-Set could look like this</u>**:

**GRIND** – Neuro-Grip push-ups
    Immediately followed by:

**DYNAMIC POWER DRILL**- Plyometric push-ups
    Immediately followed by:

**ISOMETRIC**- Lower crossover chest contraction

These three combined exercises complete one Neuro-Set. And a Neuro-Set taxes the various growth systems of the body like nothing else.

# The Kettlebell and Extreme Bodyweight Exercises— Choosing the Path of MOST Resistance

"Anything that you do to make your workout harder will be a step in the right direction."
- Mike Mentzer

There is a trend in the world of fitness to make exercise easier. The problem is that it takes resistance to build muscle and strength. Resistance is not an enemy to be feared, but rather something we should embrace. Those who choose the path of least resistance will find themselves making mediocre gains at best. The Neuro-Mass system chooses the path of most resistance. The protocols and exercises are designed to create maximum stimulation of the nervous and muscular systems. Neuro-Sets are much harder than conventional training methods. The path is constructed by using kettlebells, bodyweight exercises, or both together in Hybrid mode.

The kettlebell's unique shape causes an offset center of gravity. This places the body at a biomechanical disadvantage. As a result, the body must constantly adjust to stabilize the bell during the lift. The entire body is taxed (especially the grip, forearms, and core) by the contraction required to overcome the unique leverage of the kettlebell during the Neuro-Set. The kettlebell makes regular lifts more difficult than standard dumbbells. More resistance = more muscle.

Extreme bodyweight exercises are another tool that provides powerful resistance. While machines work on isolating the muscles, bodyweight exercises allow the body to work together as a unit. This develops your coordination and functional fitness. Extreme bodyweight exercises are challenging to all levels of trainees. I have watched athletes who could bench press over 300 pounds, who were not able to perform even one Neuro-Grip push-up. Many of the bodyweight exercises in the Neuro-Mass Program will be new to most athletes. I have hand-picked these bodyweight exercises for inclusion into the Neuro-Mass arsenal.

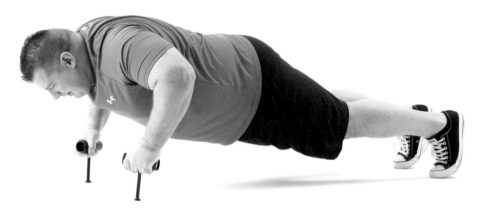

By choosing the path of most resistance through the Neuro-Mass system, there is the additional benefit of acquiring mental toughness. Mental toughness is what separates those who achieve elite performance and those who never rise above mediocrity. Without mental toughness, I would not be able to endure the feats in my strongman performances. One feat called "lifted up" is extremely taxing mentally. The stunt involves me holding two 40-pound steel crosses in a crucifix position while my wife is hanging from my head. The goal is for me to hold this position for as long as possible. The pain and discomfort requires mental endurance as much as physical endurance.

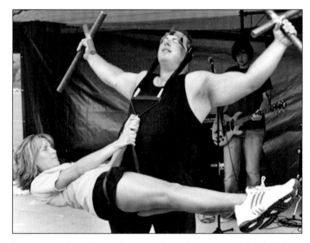

Neuro-Mass develops mental toughness by:

- Teaching the body to respond rapidly to different types of stress.
- Teaching the body to persevere through fatigue.
- Learning to embrace discomfort.
- Increasing will power and the mind-body connection through Neuro-Sets.

The path of most resistance will lead you to superior gains in mass, strength and performance.

# Breaking Down the Neuro-Set

*"There comes a moment when you have to stop revving up the car and shove it into gear"*
—David Mahoney

**N**ow that we have looked under the hood and have seen the powerful potential of Neuro-Set training, it's time to look at some performance criterion. We will break down the proper Load, Speed, Intensity, and Time during a Neuro-Set. The right combination of these logistics will allow the Neuro-Set to provide maximum gains.

## GRINDS

For kettlebells, the load should be a weight that you can perform at least eight repetitions with. The same rule applies for bodyweight exercises. Your goal during the grind portion of the Neuro-Set is to execute eight to twelve repetitions of the exercise.

**Performance Points:**
- The movement should be slow and controlled.
- Use maximum tension techniques.

# Dynamic Power Drills

The dynamic power drills will be performed for a minimum of fifteen seconds to a maximum of sixty seconds. The goal is to keep maximum speed and velocity for at least thirty seconds.

Performance Points:
- Fight the urge to slow down.
- Focus on maximum explosion.

# Isometrics

The isometric exercise portion of the Neuro-Set is performed for seven to twelve seconds. Inhale through the nose, and begin to contract and tense the muscles against the immoveable resistance. Forcefully exhale out of the mouth with pursed lips during the exercise. Your exhalation should make a hissing sound.

Performance Points:
- Do NOT hold your breath.
- Do not release tension during the exercise.
- Try to increase the contraction during the exercise.

The intensity of a Neuro-Set is high. There should be no break between exercises. Following these fundamentals is essential to Neuro-Set training.

# Athletic
# Armor-Building /
# Smart Muscle

euro-Mass allows you not to just look the part, but to become the real deal. This concept reminds me of a story told by Ravi Zacharias,

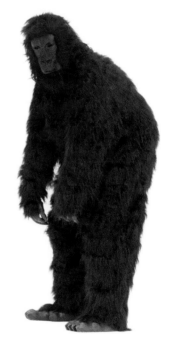

*"During some desperate times, a zoo advertised for needed help. A well-built man was rather disappointed to find that the only job left was that of impersonating a gorilla. The gorilla had died and the zoo was expecting a bunch of visitors, so they needed an imposter. Money was tight so he took the job. All went well for the first few hours but then the heat and bananas started taking their toll. As he tried to swing from one tree to another, he lost his grip and went flying into the lion's den. Immediately he started shouting, "Help! Help!" The lion then leaned over and said, "If you don't stop screaming, we will both lose our jobs."*

In the athletic jungle, too many athletes are all show and no go. Appearances can be deceiving. We have seen a great emphasis in fitness world on building the exterior without focusing on functionality. Muscle mass is important, but it shouldn't come at the cost of athleticism. That's why Neuro-Mass focuses on creating smart muscle through Athletic Armor-Building. Armor- Building is a term coined by Dan John to describe hypertrophy. The protocols in this book will develop true athletic armor, capable of taking on any challenge that is thrown at it.

Here are some of the many benefits of possessing Athletic Armor:

- Increased ability to resist injury.
- Increased strength.
- Enhanced sports performance.
- Increased work capacity.
- Increased metabolism.
- Enhanced libido.
- Increased confidence.
- Reduced stress.
- Improved ability to burn fat.
- Increased longevity of your athletic career.

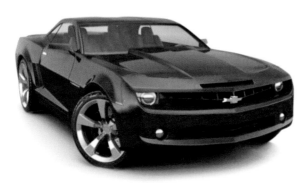

I remember when I received my first "dream car", a shiny red Camaro. It looked like the ultimate sports car for a young student. I did not take much time to check out the performance... I could just tell that it was fast. Well, it turned out after I took possession of the car, I realized it was only four cylinders. That Camaro struggled just to get up to sixty-five miles per hour! Great looking? Yes. High performance? Absolutely not! Neuro-Mass allows you to have "The Best of Both Worlds", as Sammy Hagar used to sing. By building Athletic Armor that performs as well as it looks.

# The Exercises

The Neuro-Mass system incorporates a superlative collection of kettlebell and bodyweight exercises. The following sections will provide descriptions, techniques, and performance points of all the exercises in the system. The exercises will be grouped into following categories:

- Kettlebell grinds lower body / upper body
- Kettlebell dynamic power drills lower body / upper body
- Kettlebell isometrics lower body / upper body
- Bodyweight grinds lower body / upper body
- Bodyweight dynamic power drills lower body / upper body
- Bodyweight isometrics lower body / upper body
- Neuro-Rack isometrics
- The Neuro-Burner

A thorough reading of these descriptions will help you to get the most out of the system. This section will also be a great reference tool.

## Breathing Technique for Grinds

Grinds require a version of the technique called "power breathing". This practice has been used by everyone from musicians to martial artists. In fact, I was first exposed to this method during my years of vocal performance training. We will be adding a pressurized exhalation to this technique. Power breathing is one of my secret weapons for increasing strength and power. I have blown up and burst many hot water bottles in my programs by using power breathing. The impact of the exploding bottles was so great that it would leave huge welts and cuts on my face. To remedy this, I had to actually place a piece of duct tape on each of my cheeks for protection.

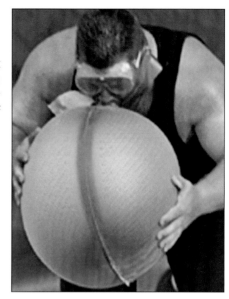

I have blown up and burst many hot water bottles in my programs by using power breathing. I had to actually place a piece of duct tape on each of my cheeks for protection.

To begin, place both of your hands on your abdomen. Allow the middle finger of each hand to touch. Now inhale through your nose into your abdomen. If you are doing this correctly, the fingers should no longer be touching. If you are not seeing your hands separate, you are "chest breathing". Once you have inhaled into your abdomen {pressurization}, tighten the abdominal muscles.

Now place your tongue against your teeth and forcefully hiss out through pursed lips. You have just completed a power breath. This technique allows you to keep pressure and tension in your core while lifting. Power breathing will increase your ability to handle the heavy loads required in Neuro-Mass.

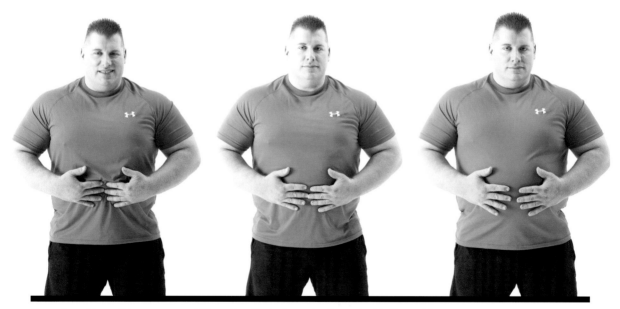

Power breathing will increase your ability to handle the heavy loads required in Neuro-Mass.

# Kettlebell Grinds Lower Body

## The Double Kettlebell Front Squat

The kettlebell squat and its variations will build massive strength in the lower body. In order to execute a kettlebell front squat, the kettlebells must first be in the rack position. This is accomplished by cleaning the kettlebells from the floor.

Begin by setting two kettlebells a few inches in front of your big toe. The handles should form a v shape. This not only helps in the performance of the clean, but is essential for shoulder health. While keeping your back flat, hinge at your hips and grasp the kettlebells. The thumbs should be pointing toward your body. Hike the bells backward through the legs.

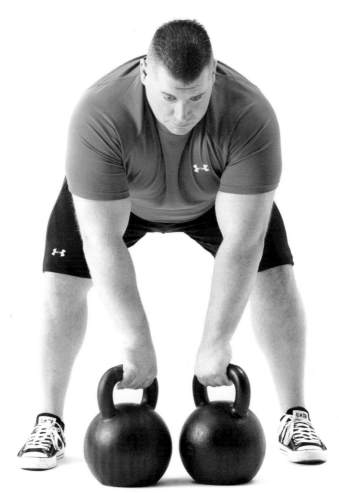

Double kettlebell
clean beginning

Now, reverse the movement by using your hips to propel the bells forward and upward. As the hips explode forward, bend the elbows so that your hands rotate the bells around your wrist. Tighten the core to prepare the body to absorb the impact. Keep your elbows tight to your sides. The bells are now in the rack position.

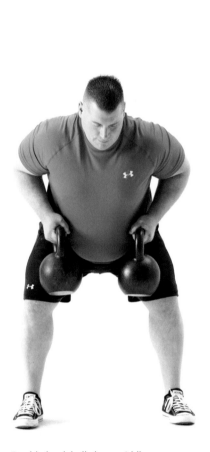

Double kettlebell clean middle

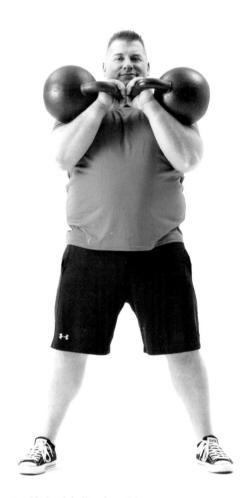

Double kettlebell rack position

From the rack position, bring your hands together so that the bells are resting on the chest. The feet should be set at slightly beyond shoulder width apart. Inhale, and with maximum tension begin to pull yourself down into the bottom position of the squat. Now, keeping maximum tension, squeeze the glute muscles, push your chest out, and drive up to the starting position. Keep tension and pressure in the core by using the power breathing exhalation technique on the second part of the lift.

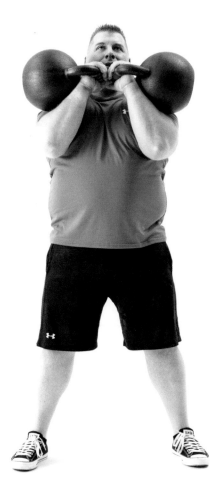

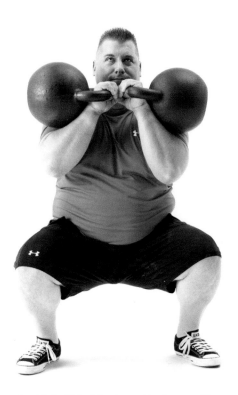

Double kettlebell front squat rack position

Double kettlebell front squat bottom position

# The Double Kettlebell Lateral Step Squat

Lateral movement is a key to developing smart mass. Most athletic competitions require some form of lateral movement. This exercise also encourages hip mobility, body awareness, and balance.

To begin, clean the bells into the rack position. With elbows tight to the body, bring the hands together so that the bells are resting on the chest. The feet are set slightly inside the shoulder length apart. Inhale with maximum pressurization, raise the right foot around six inches in the air while simultaneously pushing laterally with the left foot. Absorb the impact with right foot as you pull yourself down into the squat position. Now, with chest high, and tensed glutes, drive upwards and laterally by pushing off of the right foot. The right foot will come off the ground again around six inches as you are returning to the starting position. Remember to power breath to keep tension on the core. Now, repeat the movement in the opposite direction. This exercise takes some time to master.

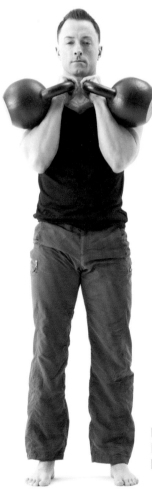

Double kettlebell
lateral step squat
beginning position

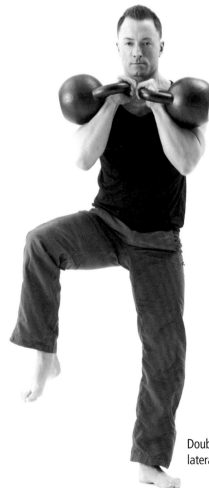

Double kettlebell
lateral movement

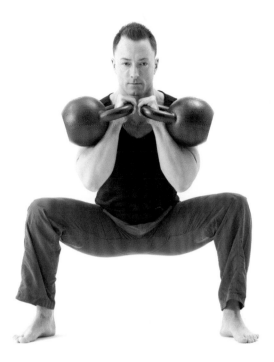

**Performance Point:** When moving laterally to the right, make sure that the left foot stays planted. When moving laterally to the left, the right foot should stay planted. The double kettlebell lateral step squat can take your body to new levels of athleticism.

Double kettlebell lateral step squat bottom position

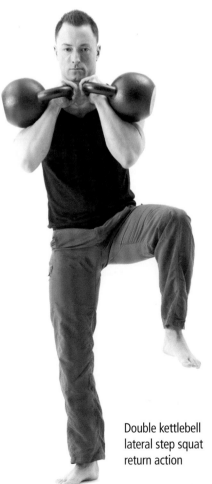

Double kettlebell lateral step squat return action

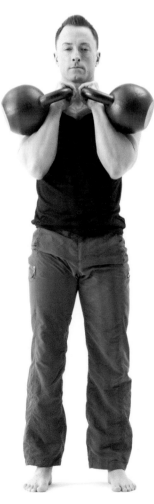

Double kettlebell lateral step squat finishing position

## The Double Kettlebell Front Elevation Lunge

For this exercise you will need a step that is six to ten inches in height. The front foot will be placed on the step increasing the range of motion, stretch, and muscle recruitment. Place the step two or more feet in front of your body. Clean two kettlebells into the rack position. The elbows should be tight against the sides of the body while the bells rest on the chest. Step forward so that one foot is resting on the platform. The front foot should be in complete contact with the step. The rear heel will be off the floor. The front knee is partially bent.

Now, inhale and create tension and pressure within the body. Lower the body toward the floor. To ascend, push hard with the elevated foot driving back up to the starting position. Remember to power breathe on the way up.

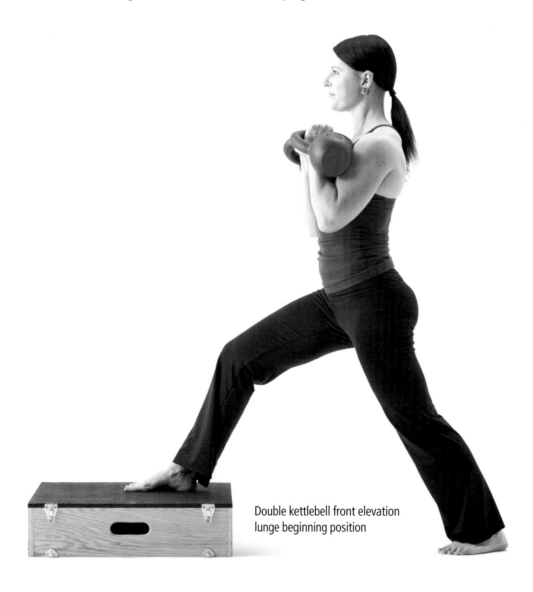

Double kettlebell front elevation lunge beginning position

22

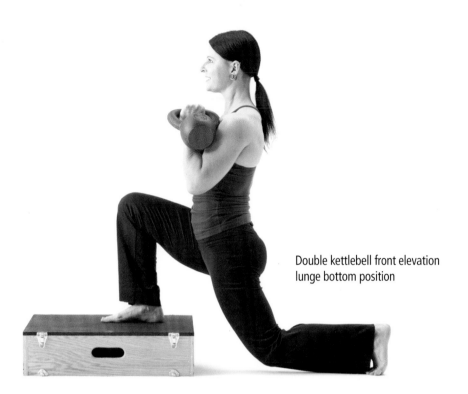

Double kettlebell front elevation
lunge bottom position

**Performance Points:** Make sure to
keep the back straight during this
exercise. Fight the urge to lean
forward. Finish all the repetitions on
one leg before switching to the other
leg. Because of the extreme range of
motion involved in this exercise, you
should use lighter kettlebells.

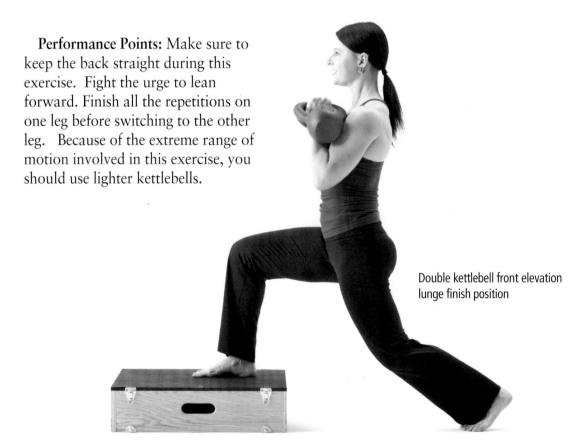

Double kettlebell front elevation
lunge finish position

# The Double Kettlebell Rear Elevation Lunge

Just as in the previous exercise, you will need a step or platform six to ten inches in height. This movement really taxes the quads. Place the step behind you. Clean the kettlebells into the proper rack position. Lift one foot behind you until it is in contact with the top of the step. The heel of the elevated foot should not be touching the step. Pushing off with the rear foot, step the front foot forward. The knee of the front leg should be partially bent. This is the beginning position of the exercise.

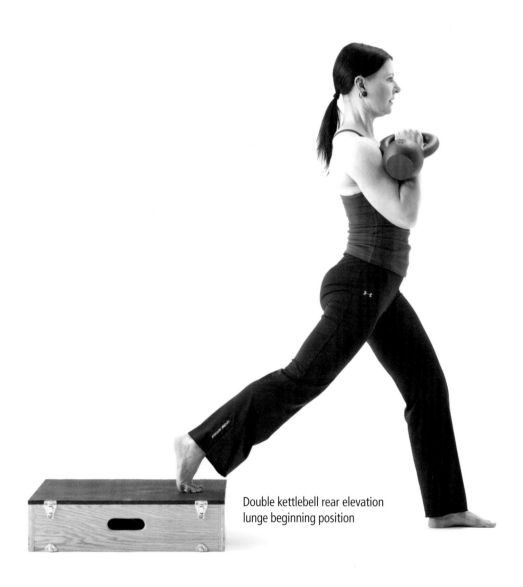

Double kettlebell rear elevation lunge beginning position

**Performance Points:** Keep your chest high and back straight. Complete all of the required repetitions on one leg before switching to the other leg. The balance and range of motion make this a very challenging exercise. It would be wise to use a lighter pair of kettlebells.

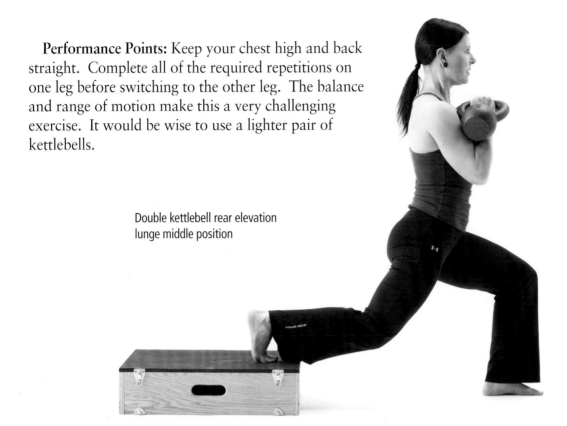

Double kettlebell rear elevation lunge middle position

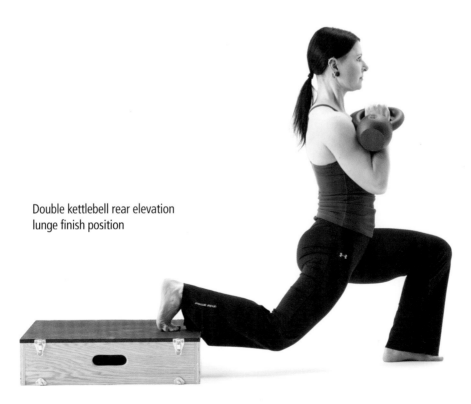

Double kettlebell rear elevation lunge finish position

# The Double Kettlebell Wide Squat

Clean a pair of kettlebells to the rack position. Now, separate your feet so that they are wider than shoulder width apart. Your toes should be slightly pointed outward. Inhale, and create tension and pressurize the core. Actively pull yourself into the bottom position of the squat. Pause for a moment, then squeeze the glutes hard, as you drive up into the starting position. Remember to power breathe on the way up.

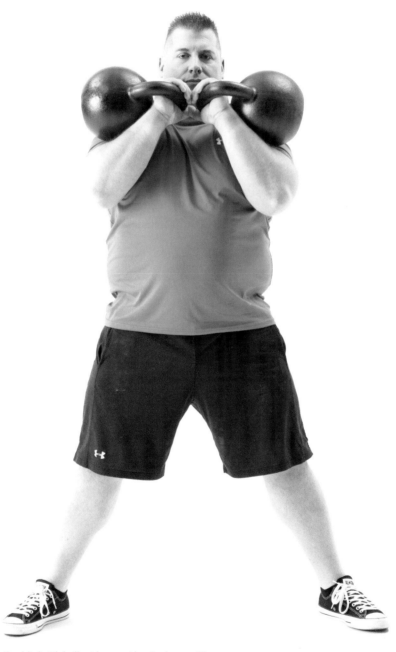

Double kettlebell wide squat beginning position

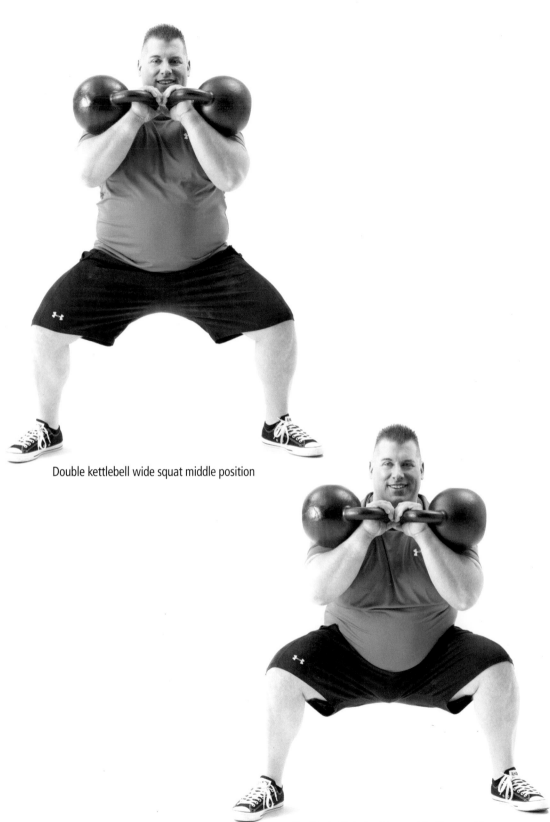

Double kettlebell wide squat middle position

Double kettlebell wide squat bottom position

# The Double Kettlebell Ballet Squat

To begin clean a pair of medium weight kettlebells to the rack position. The elbows should be tight against the body as the bells rest on the chest. Bring the heels together with toes pointing out at a 45 degree angle. Inhale and pressurize your core. Now slowly lower into the bottom position of the squat. The heels should both come up off the floor during the lowering part of the exercise. The glutes should be tensed during the descending and ascending portion of the lift. Now using the power breath exhalation technique, drive straight upwards pushing off from your toes until you reach the starting position.

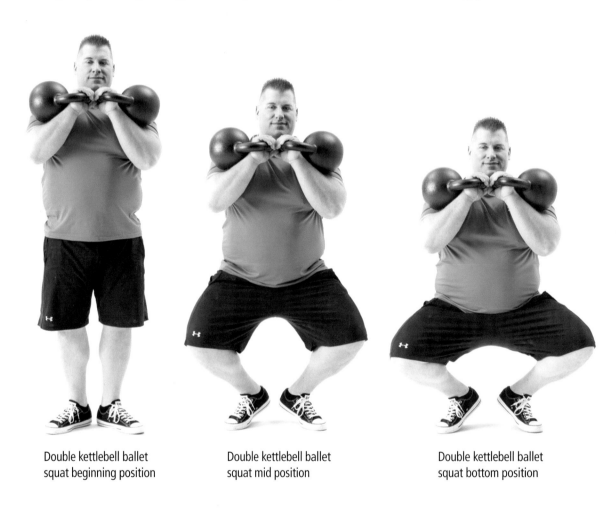

Double kettlebell ballet
squat beginning position

Double kettlebell ballet
squat mid position

Double kettlebell ballet
squat bottom position

This exercise will not only develop your strength, but your balance as well.

**Performance Point:** Using lighter kettlebells for this exercise is essential due to the unique leverage and balance challenges.

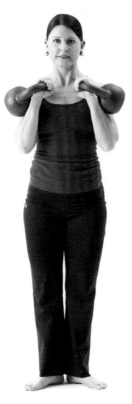
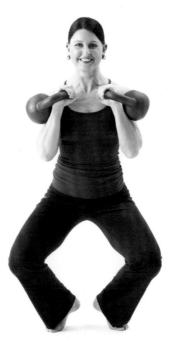
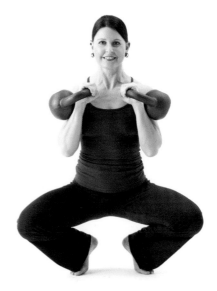

Double kettlebell ballet
squat beginning position

Double kettlebell ballet
squat mid position

Double kettlebell ballet
squat bottom position

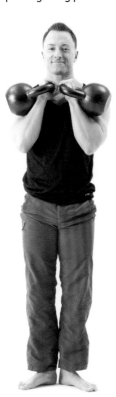
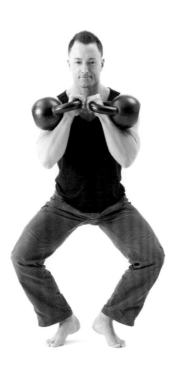
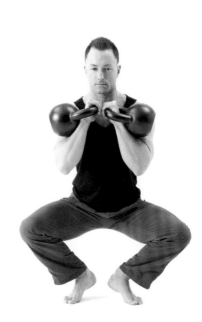

# The Double Kettlebell Sumo Deadlift

Begin by placing two heavy kettlebells between your legs. Your feet should be wider than shoulder length apart. Inhale as you squat down. Now, grasp the kettlebells and squeeze the handles. Driving your feet through the floor, squeeze your glutes and rise to the top position. Remember to power breathe. Inhale, create maximum tension and squat down to the bottom position. When the kettlebells touch the floor, immediately start the ascent for the next repetition.

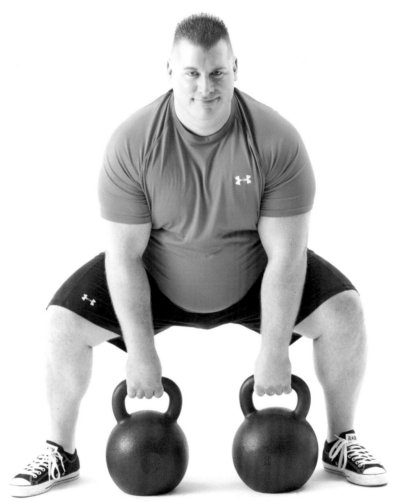

Double kettlebell sumo deadlift beginning position

The double kettlebell sumo deadlift is a great all around strength builder. It works all the muscles from the neck on down.

**Performance Point:** Don't look down at the kettlebells while performing the action portion of this exercise. Keep your back straight

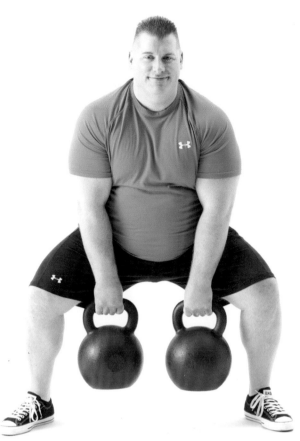

Double kettlebell sumo deadlift middle position

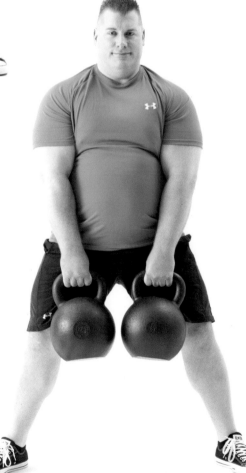

Double kettlebell sumo
deadlift finish position

## The Double Kettlebell Suitcase Deadlift

Begin by placing two heavy kettlebells between your legs. Your feet should be wider than shoulder length apart. Inhale as you squat down. Now, grasp the kettlebells and squeeze the handles. Driving your feet through the floor, squeeze your glutes and rise to the top position. Remember to power breathe. Inhale, create maximum tension and squat down to the bottom position. When the kettlebells touch the floor, immediately start the ascent for the next repetition.

This is a great way to build a powerful core and a strong set of wheels.

**Performance Point:** keep your focus straight ahead. Don't round your back.

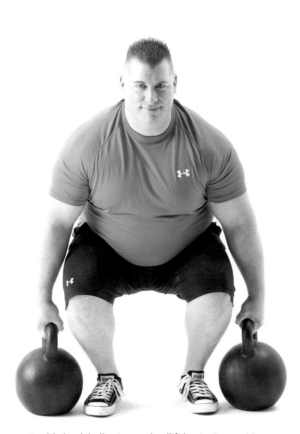

Double kettlebell suitcase deadlift beginning position

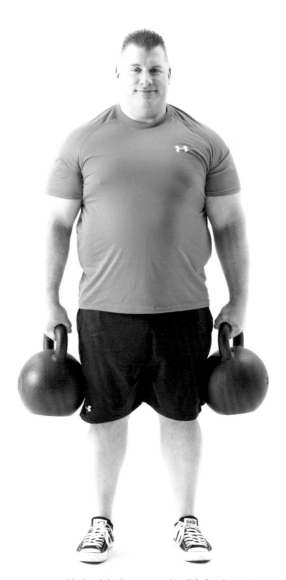

Double kettlebell suitcase deadlift finish position

# The Double Kettlebell Calf Raise

Place a heavy kettlebell on the outside of each foot. Squat down and grasp the kettlebells. Stand up, and step onto a small platform that is 4 to 6 inches high. Only the front half of your feet should remain on the platform. Now, squeeze your calf muscles and raise your heels straight up into the air. You should feel a strong contraction in the calves. Now lower your heels until you feel a slight stretch. Repeat the movement for the required repetitions.

**Performance Point:** For variety you may point the toes outward during this exercise to hit the calves from a different angle.

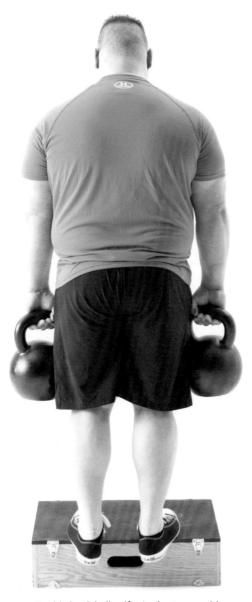

Double kettlebell calf raise bottom position

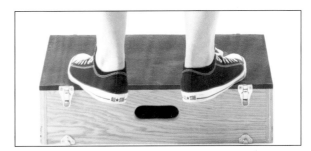

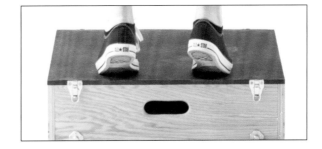

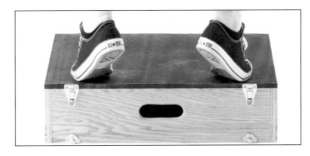

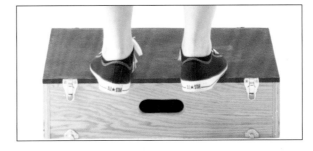

# Kettlebell Grinds Upper Body

## Double Kettlebell Overhead Press

The double kettlebell press is one of the best exercises to build size and strength in the upper body. To begin, clean the kettlebells to your chest. Now, inhale and crush the handles while creating full body tension. Begin to slowly press the bells overhead using the power in your lats and triceps. Keeping your chest out at the top of the exercise, the bells should lock out slightly toward the back of your head. Power exhale through the upward pressing motion. Pause before lowering the bells.

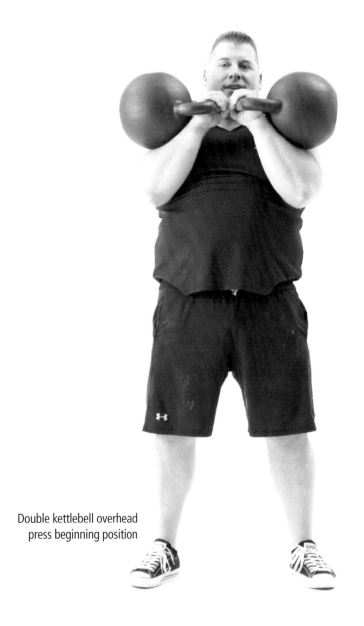

Double kettlebell overhead
press beginning position

To descend, inhale and actively pull the bells down to the rack position using your lats. Exhale at the bottom portion of the lift. To create maximum tension, squeeze the glutes during the exercise.

**Performance Points:** Don't bend the wrists while pressing. Recruit power from the lats, glutes and core.

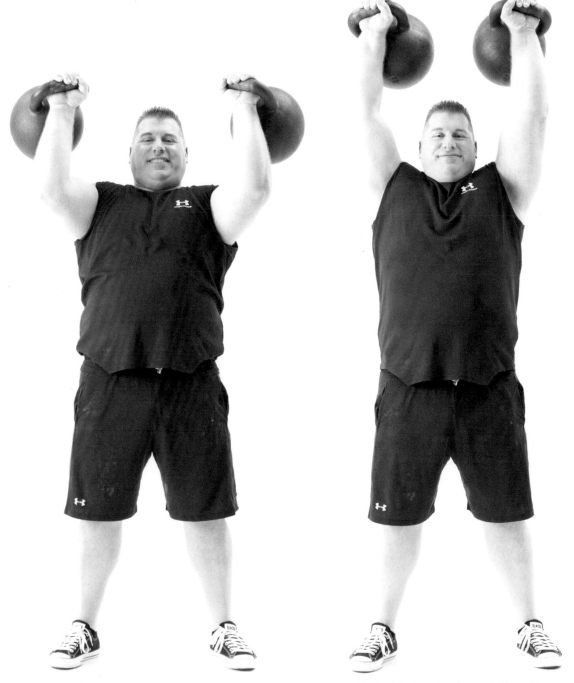

Double kettlebell overhead press middle position

Double kettlebell overhead press finish position

# Double Kettlebell Bottoms Up Overhead Press

This is a great exercise that stimulates hypertrophy because of the extreme stress it places on the musculature. This lift has great carryover potential for strongmen, as it simulates the log press. My technique for this lift may be different from others.

To start, place two medium weight kettlebells in between your feet. Inhale, hinge at the hips, reach down and crush the kettlebell handles. Now, swing the bells backward and through the legs. Crush the handles during the backward swing. Reverse the movement by leading with the hips. Bend your elbows on the way up as you clean the kettlebells to the bottoms up clean position. You may exhale after the bells are in the clean position. Inhale, keeping maximum tension, press the bells overhead. Power breathe throughout the movement.

Inhale, and actively pull the bells down to the starting position.

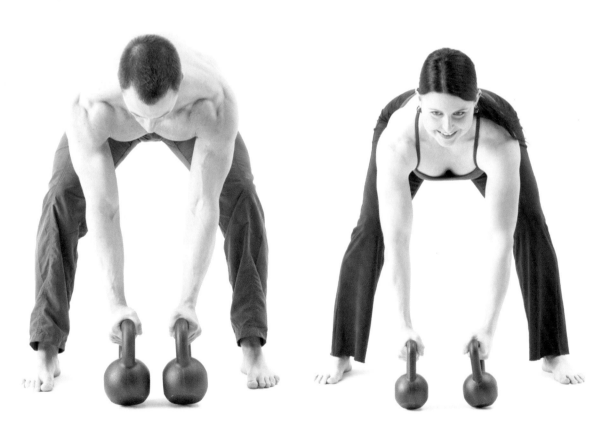

Double kettlebell bottoms up overhead press beginning position

**Performance Points:** Because of the difficulty of this exercise, it is a good idea to start with lighter kettlebells. Focus on maximum tension to avoid power leakages in the body.

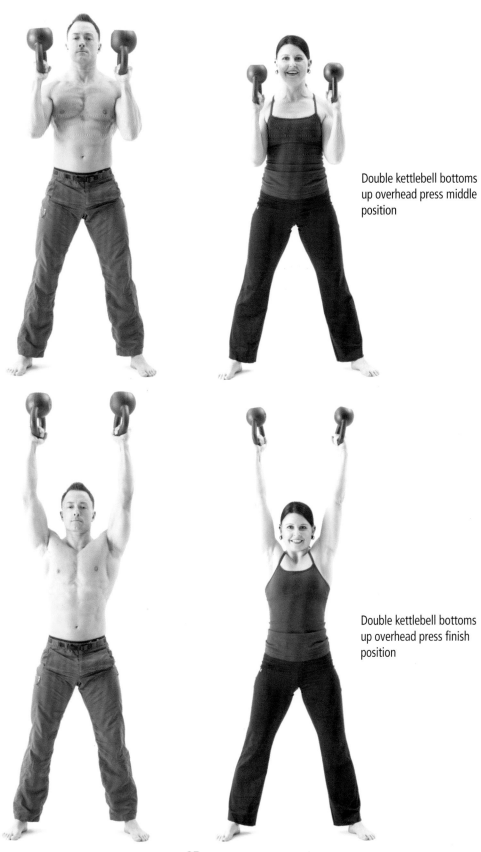

Double kettlebell bottoms up overhead press middle position

Double kettlebell bottoms up overhead press finish position

# Double Kettlebell Crucifix

This is an excellent exercise to create massive shoulders and bulletproof wrists. To perform the crucifix properly requires tension and control.

Begin by performing a double kettlebell bottoms up clean. Following the correct steps outlined earlier, press the kettlebells overhead. Now, inhale and turn your palms facing forward. Pack your shoulders and lower the kettlebells into the crucifix position. Power breathe, and slowly raise the bells back overhead.

**Performance Points:** You must use light kettlebells in this exercise to avoid injury. Make sure that you perform this exercise very slowly. Make sure not to bend your wrists.

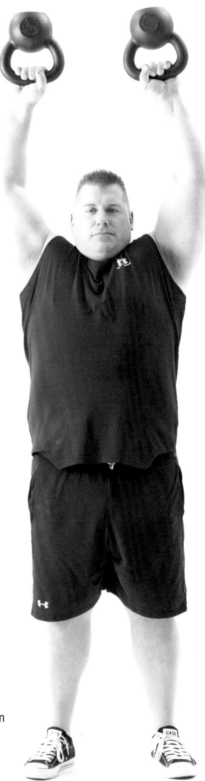

Double kettlebell crucifix beginning position

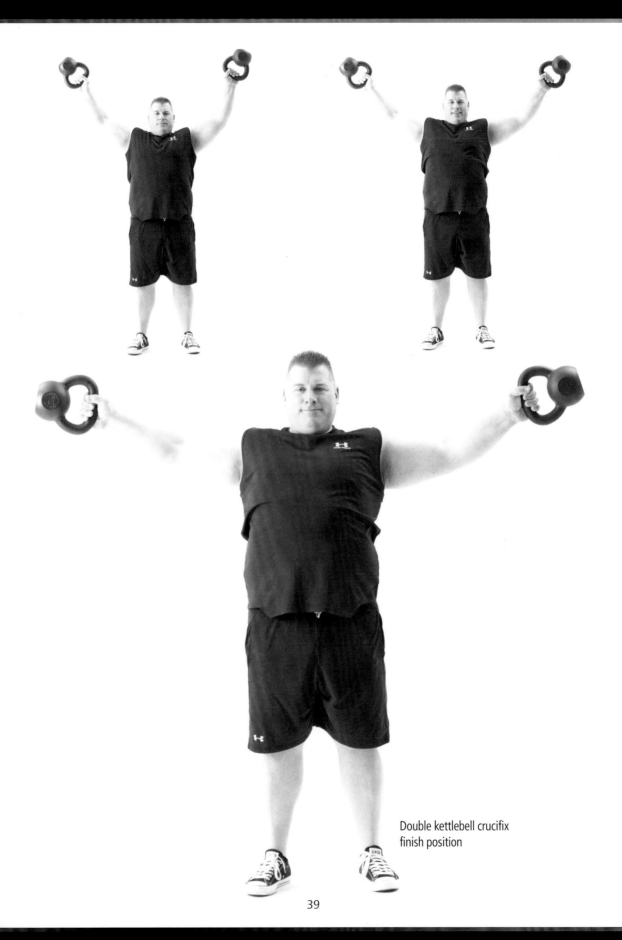

Double kettlebell crucifix
finish position

# Double Kettlebell Bench Press

This is a superior exercise to build a big chest. The groove that kettlebells follow really stimulates the pectoral muscles. To begin, place a sturdy bench behind you. Inhale and bring two kettlebells to the proper rack position. Slowly, sit backwards until you are seated, exhale. Inhale, and roll back onto the bench. Turn your elbows out so that your palms are facing forward. Your forearms should form a vertical line toward the ceiling. Now, press the bells in an upward arcing manner. The arms should form a straight line at the top of the movement. Power exhale through the pressing motion. Inhale, and actively pull the bells down to the starting position.

Once you have completed the required repetitions, bring your elbows back tight to the sides of your body. Roll up to the seated position. Inhale, stand up, lower the bells to the floor.

**Performance Points:**
Practice sitting backward onto the bench without the bells, for safety.

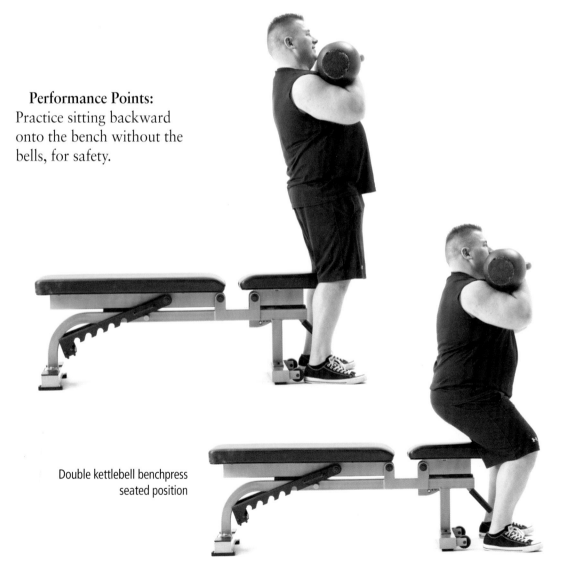

Double kettlebell benchpress
seated position

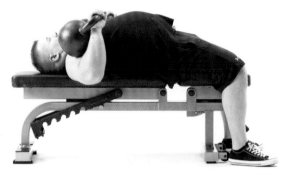

Double kettlebell benchpress prone position

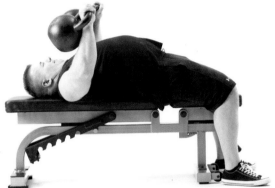

Double kettlebell benchpress middle position

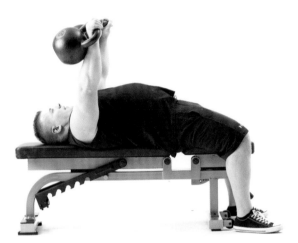

Double kettlebell benchpress finish position

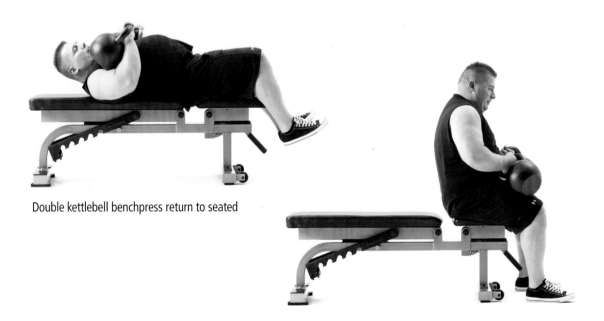

Double kettlebell benchpress return to seated

## Double Kettlebell Incline Bench Press

Follow the bench press guidelines, but use a bench set at a thirty degree angle instead of a flat bench.

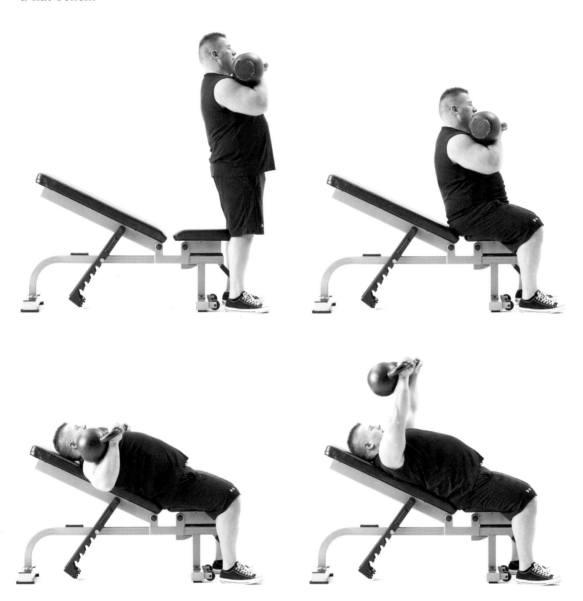

## Double Kettlebell Bench Flyes

Since the kettlebells feature an offset center of gravity, they create resistance during the full range of motion of this exercise. The result of this resistance is a larger and stronger chest / shoulder girdle. Before attempting this exercise, make sure there is a sturdy bench behind you. Inhale and clean two kettlebells to the rack position. Squat backwards until you are seated on the bench, exhale. Inhale, as you slowly roll back into the supine position, exhale. Now inhale as you press both kettlebells straight up. Exhale and turn your palms facing each other. Inhale and pressurize the core, and slowly lower the bells until you feel a slight stretch in the chest. Crushing the handles, raise the bells to the starting position while power breathing.

After completing the required number of repetitions, lower the bells to your chest keeping your elbows tight to your sides. Inhale, and roll back up into the seated position, exhale. Inhale, pressurizing your core, and stand up. Now lower the bells to the floor.

**Performance Points:**
Because this exercise moves through such an extreme range of motion, it is recommended to start with a lighter pair of kettlebells. Also, do not go beyond a slight stretch in the lower position of this exercise.

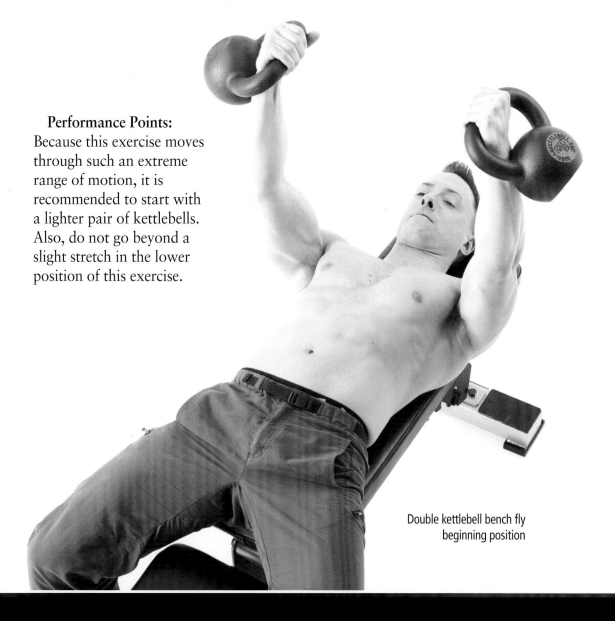

Double kettlebell bench fly
beginning position

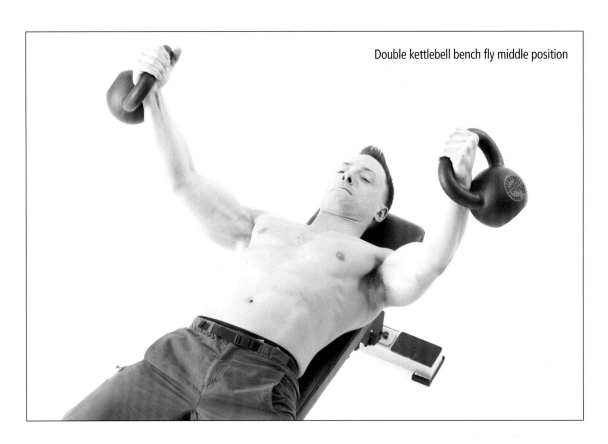

Double kettlebell bench fly middle position

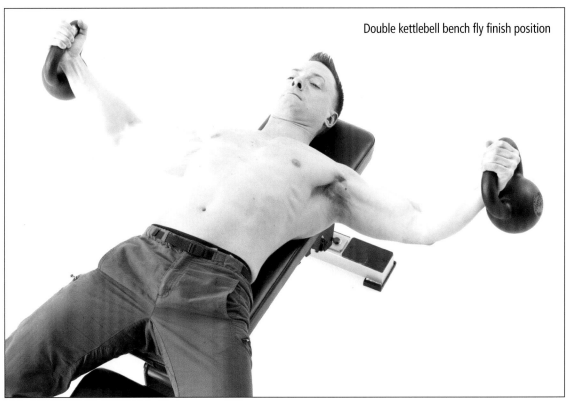

Double kettlebell bench fly finish position

# Double Kettlebell Bent Over Row

To bring true balance and power to the upper body the back muscles cannot be neglected. The double kettlebell row will build a thick muscular back.

To begin, place two heavy kettlebells just inside of your instep. The kettlebell handles should form an upside down V. Hinging at the hips and keeping your back straight, sit backwards until your hands can reach the bells. Inhale, crush the handles, and row the bells to the top position. Lead with the elbows and squeeze the shoulder blades together as you are rowing. Exhale, inhale and slowly lower the bells. Repeat for the required amount of reps.

**Performance Points:** Do not round your back. Practice hinging at the hips to make sure you have good form.

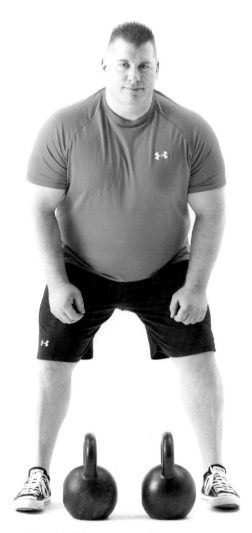

Double kettlebell bent over row beginning position

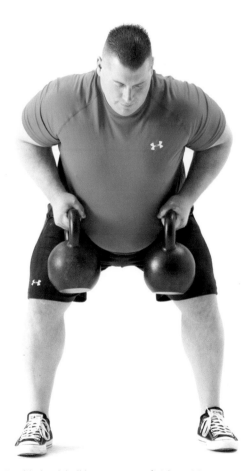

Double kettlebell bent over row finish position

# Double Kettlebell Twist

Start by cleaning a pair of kettlebells to the rack position. Your feet should be about shoulder width apart. Now, keeping your feet grounded, slowly twist your torso to the right and then to the left. The movement should be very slow and controlled. Make sure to keep your core pressurized during this exercise. Repeat the movement for the required number of repetitions.

**Performance Points:** Tightening the glutes will help you maintain proper technique with this exercise.

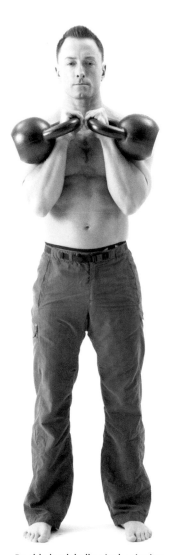
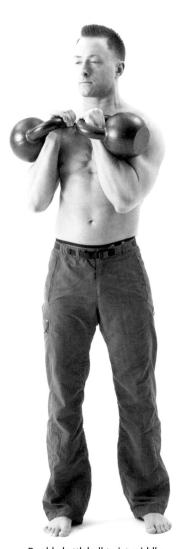
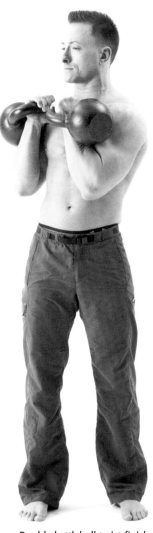

| Double kettlebell twist beginning | Double kettlebell twist middle | Double kettlebell twist finish |

## How to Modify the Double Kettlebell Grinds

If you are not able to use a pair of kettlebells on these exercises they can be modified. Simply grasp a single kettlebell by the horns and hold it at chest level. Make sure to keep the elbows tight to your sides. To increase the difficulty and leverage factor, hold the kettlebell farther away from your body. This is a great way to incrementally progress toward being able to hold a pair of kettlebells..

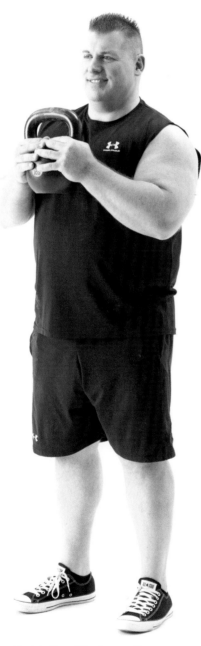

Kettlebell modification position one

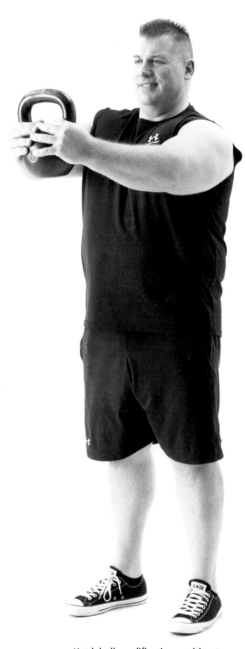

Kettlebell modification position two

## The Kettlebell Crush Press

Place a kettlebell on the floor in the inverted position so that the handle is facing downward. Now, grasp the kettlebell with your palms and step your feet back so that you are in a push-up position. Maintain your balance by crushing the bell as hard as you can. Slowly lower your upper body downward until the bell is almost touching your chest. Now, reverse the movement to the starting position and repeat the exercise for the required amount of repetitions.

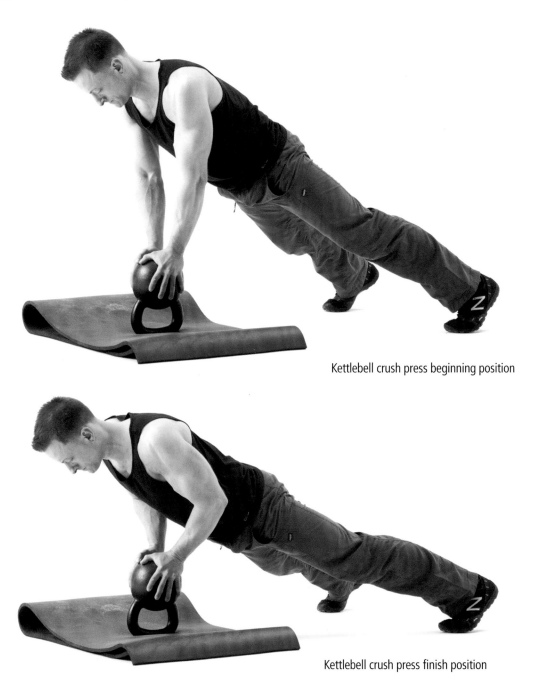

Kettlebell crush press beginning position

Kettlebell crush press finish position

# The Kettlebell Crush Pull Up

Begin by attaching a light kettlebell to a pull up bar using a daisy chain. Grasp the kettlebell with your palms crushing it as hard as you can. Now, slowly begin to pull yourself upward until the kettlebell is at chest level. Slowly lower yourself down to the beginning position and repeat the exercise for the required amount of repetitions. If the kettlebell crush pull up is too difficult, you may attach the kettlebell to a lat pulldown machine and get the same effect.

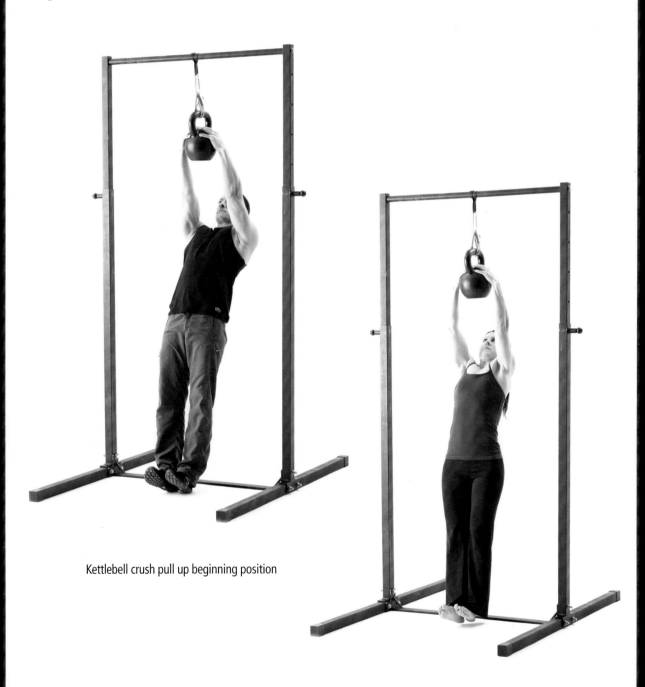

Kettlebell crush pull up beginning position

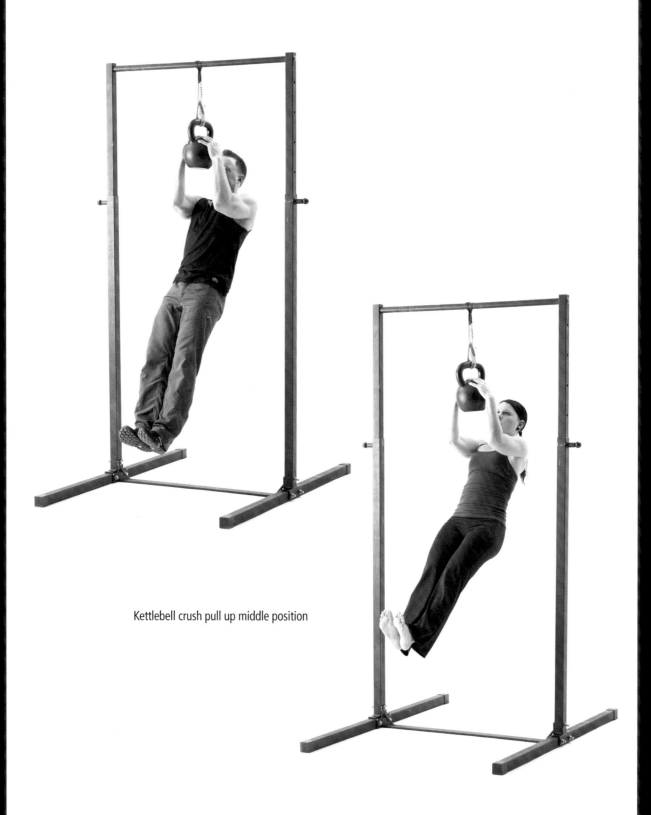

Kettlebell crush pull up middle position

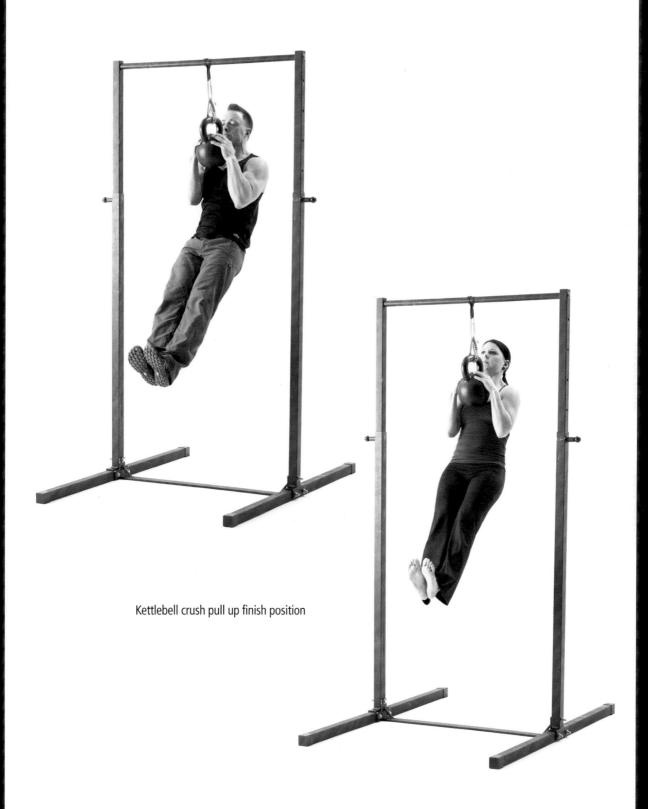

Kettlebell crush pull up finish position

# The Kettlebell Crush Inverted Row

    Start by attaching a light kettlebell with a daisy chain to a low hanging bar. Lay down on your back below the kettlebell. Grasp the kettlebell with your palms and crush it as hard as you can.  Now, slowly pull yourself upward driving your elbows backward and squeezing your shoulder blades together. Reverse the movement by slowly lowering yourself to the beginning position. Repeat the exercise for the required amount of repetitions.

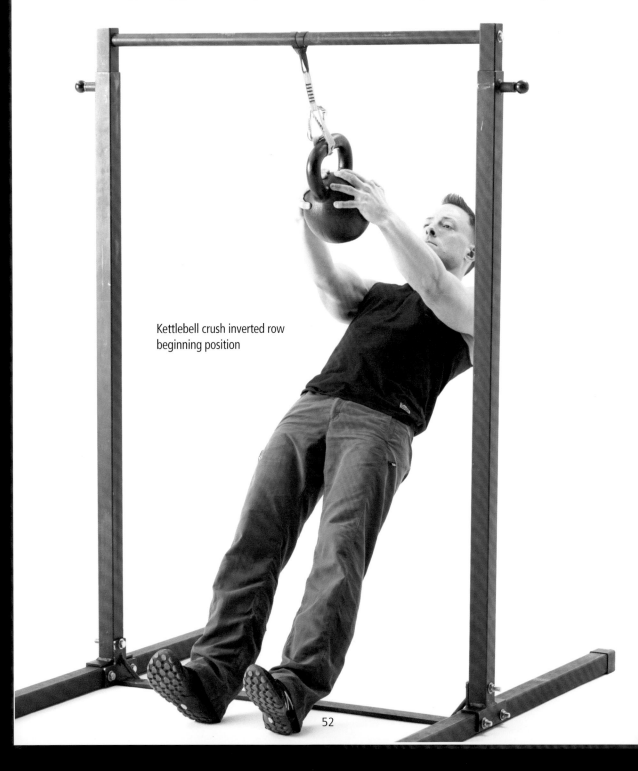

Kettlebell crush inverted row
beginning position

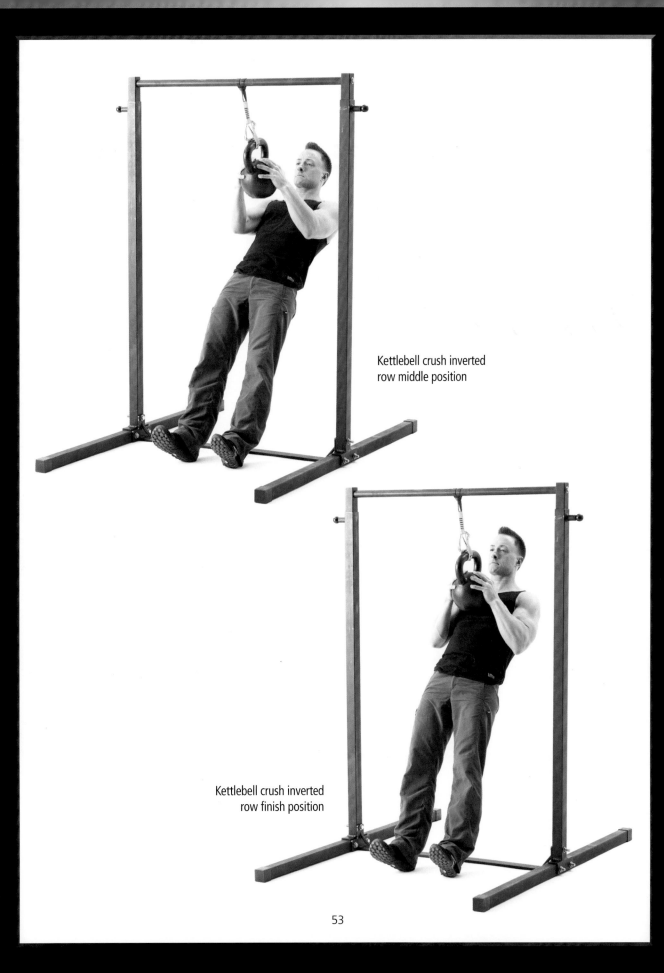

Kettlebell crush inverted
row middle position

Kettlebell crush inverted
row finish position

53

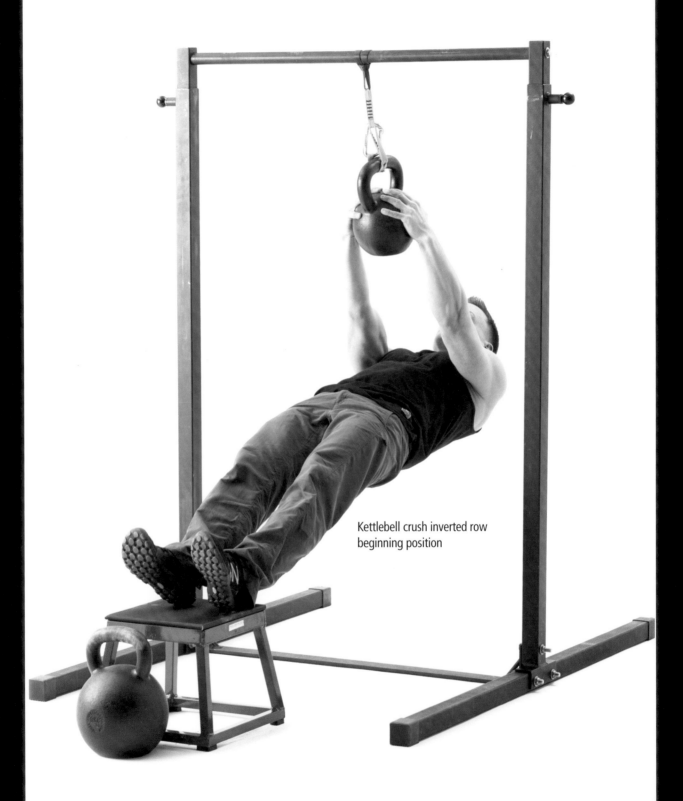

Kettlebell crush inverted row
beginning position

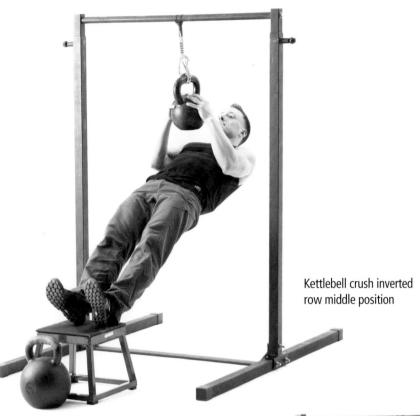

Kettlebell crush inverted
row middle position

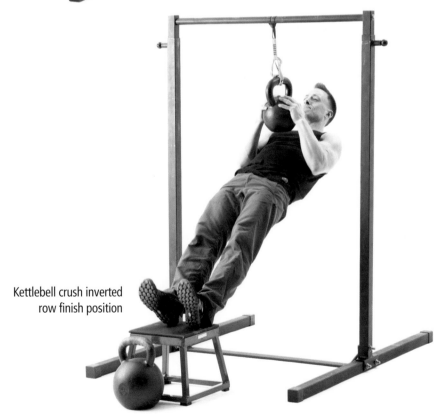

Kettlebell crush inverted
row finish position

## The Kettlebell Claw Curl

This is a grip exercise that will bring tremendous form development. Pick up a kettlebell in front of you using only the tips of your fingers. Now with maximum tension, slowly curl your fingers into your palm. Pause for a moment, and slowly uncurl your fingers until the bell is in the starting position. Repeat the exercise for the required amount of reps.

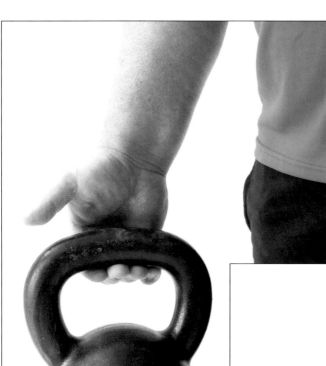

Kettlebell claw curl beginning position

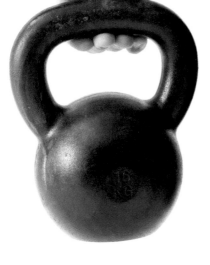

Kettlebell claw curl finish position

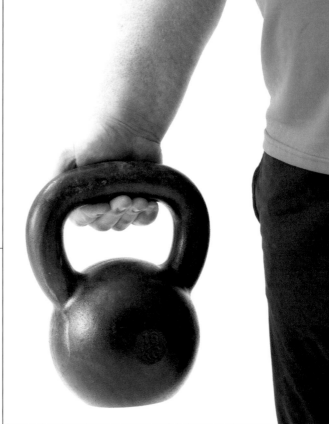

56

# Kettlebell Dynamic Power Drills, Lower Body

## Double Kettlebell Deadlift Mule Kick Combo

This dynamic movement begins by placing two heavy kettlebells in front of you. Grasp the kettlebells and lift them to a standing position. Now, slowly lower the bells to the floor. As soon as the bells touch the floor, crush the handles, lean forward and explosively kick both legs up into the air. When your toes hit the ground, jump both legs forward to the starting position. Repeat this movement for the required time.

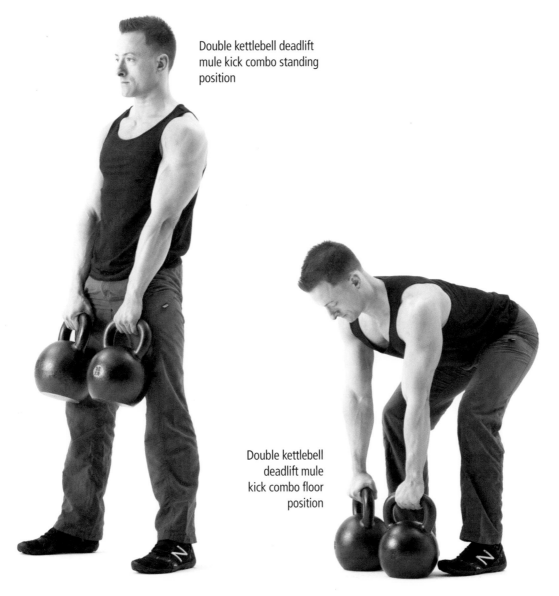

Double kettlebell deadlift mule kick combo standing position

Double kettlebell deadlift mule kick combo floor position

**Performance Points:** This exercise can be technically demanding. You may want to practice without kettlebells to find the right rhythm and technique.

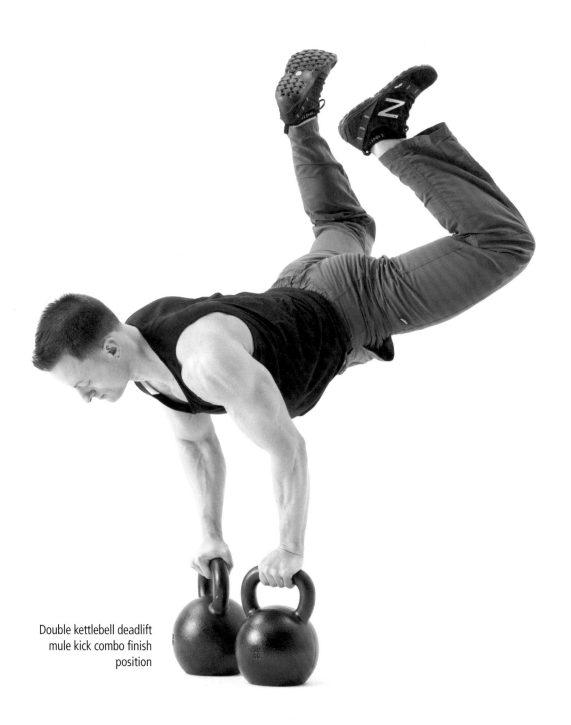

Double kettlebell deadlift mule kick combo finish position

# Single Kettlebell Explosive Lunge

Grasp a single kettlebell by the horns and hold at chest level. Keeping the elbows tight to your sides and your back straight, step one leg behind you until you are into a lunge position. Now, explosively drive your body straight into the air. While airborne, switch legs so that the rear leg is now in the front lunge position. Make sure to do this exercise as rapidly as possible. You will develop great quickness and speed that has great carryover to many other athletic activities. Repeat this exercise for the required amount of time.

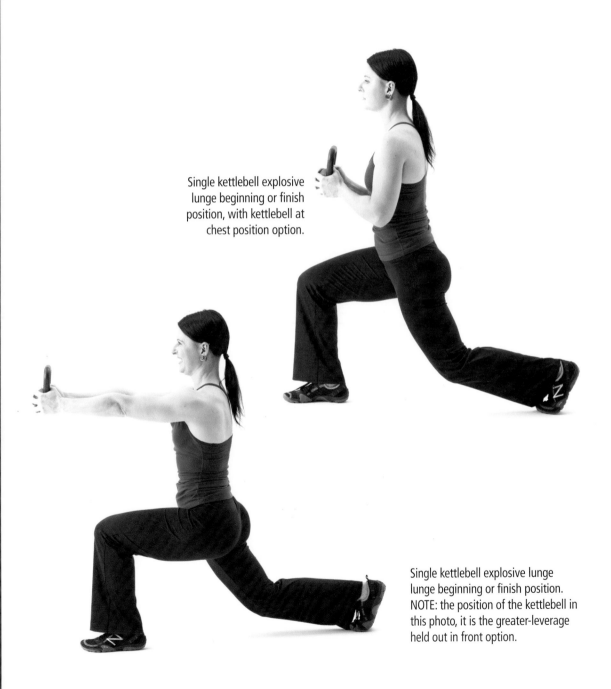

Single kettlebell explosive lunge beginning or finish position, with kettlebell at chest position option.

Single kettlebell explosive lunge lunge beginning or finish position. NOTE: the position of the kettlebell in this photo, it is the greater-leverage held out in front option.

**Performance Points:** Make sure not to lean forward during this exercise. Do not lunge too deeply, because you will compromise your speed and explosiveness.

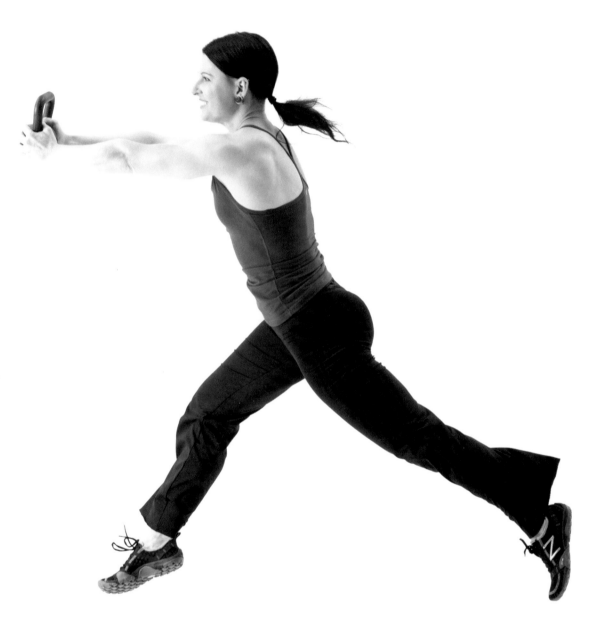

Single kettlebell explosive lunge airborne position. NOTE: photo shows the arms extended version of the exercise

# Double Kettlebell Outside The Legs Swing

This exercise builds tremendous jumping power. In fact, the form is the same as the standing long jump. Grasp two heavy kettlebells to a standing position where they are hanging at your sides. Now, hinging at the hips, hike the kettlebells behind you. To reverse the movement, propel the kettlebells forward by explosively driving with the hips and squeezing the glutes. The bells should rise to about chest level. Make sure that the arms are guiding the kettlebells outside of the legs.

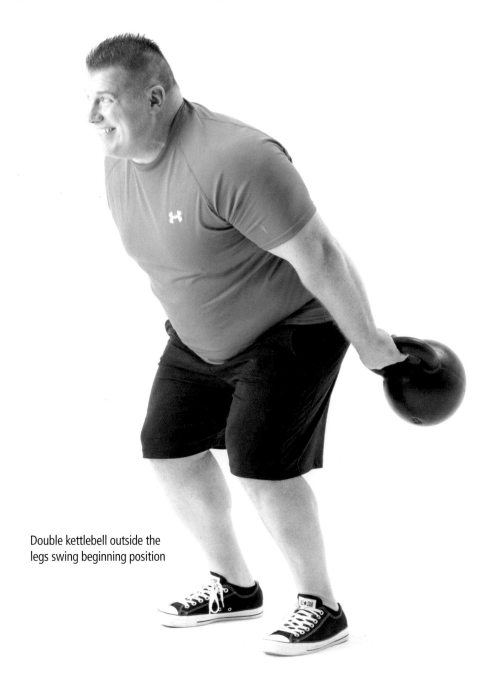

Double kettlebell outside the legs swing beginning position

**Performance Points:** Make sure to be aware of the bells at all times during this exercise, you don't want to have a kettlebell hit your knees.

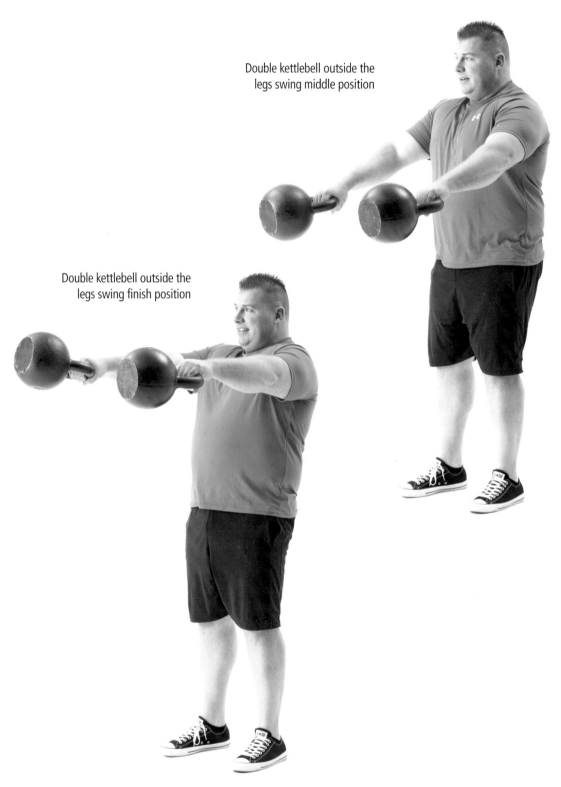

Double kettlebell outside the legs swing middle position

Double kettlebell outside the legs swing finish position

# Single Kettlebell Anchor Sprints

This exercise creates a biomechanical disadvantage and will build tremendous athleticism. Pick up a light kettlebell by the horns and bring it to chest level. Lower your hands until they are crushing the sides of the kettlebell. Press your arms straight forward and lock your elbows. Now, begin an all-out sprint. You will find that it is difficult to focus on crushing the kettlebell and sprinting at the same time. This type of training makes your nervous system smarter. Continue to sprint for the required amount of time.

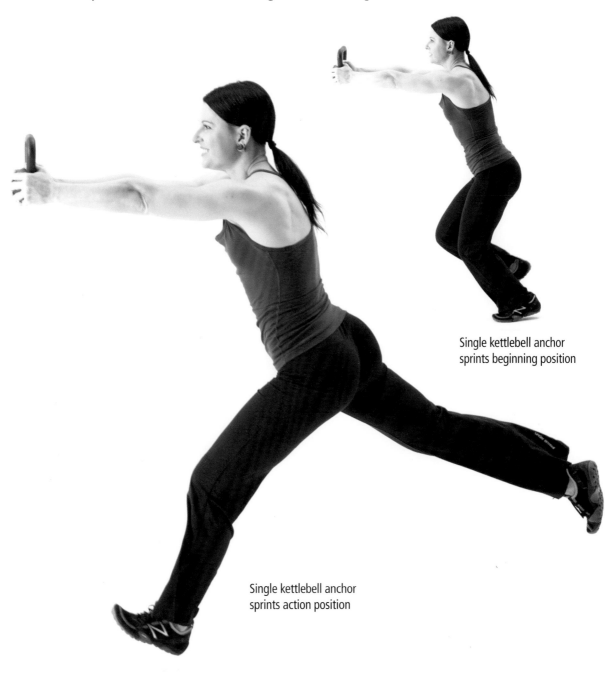

Single kettlebell anchor sprints beginning position

Single kettlebell anchor sprints action position

# Kettlebell High Pull To Catch Squat

This exercise combines upper and lower body movement. There's a tremendous loading effect, similar to plyometrics, which takes place when this exercise is done correctly. Place a heavy kettlebell in between your legs and squat down and grasp the handle with both hands. Now, driving your feet through the floor explosively pull the kettlebell straight up with a shrugging motion. As the kettlebell reaches chest height, release the handles and allow the bell to be airborne. Catch the kettlebell by crushing the sides with your hands. The elbows should be tight to the body.

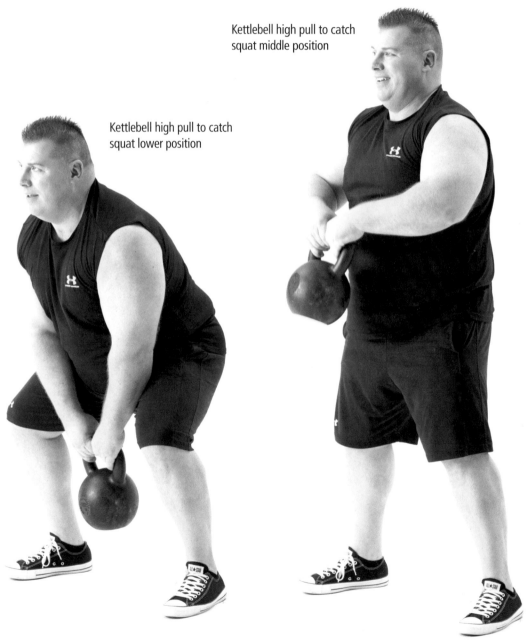

Kettlebell high pull to catch squat middle position

Kettlebell high pull to catch squat lower position

64

Immediately drop into a front squat. At the bottom of the squat, drive back up out of the hole to the standing position. From the standing position, let the bell slide through the hands until you can catch the handle. Let the bell drop down to the starting position. Repeat the exercise for the required amount of time.

**Performance Point:** Practice the catching portion of this exercise with a lighter kettlebell until you have the technique down. To get the loading effect, make sure to squat immediately after you catch the bell. Don't pull the bell into your chin.

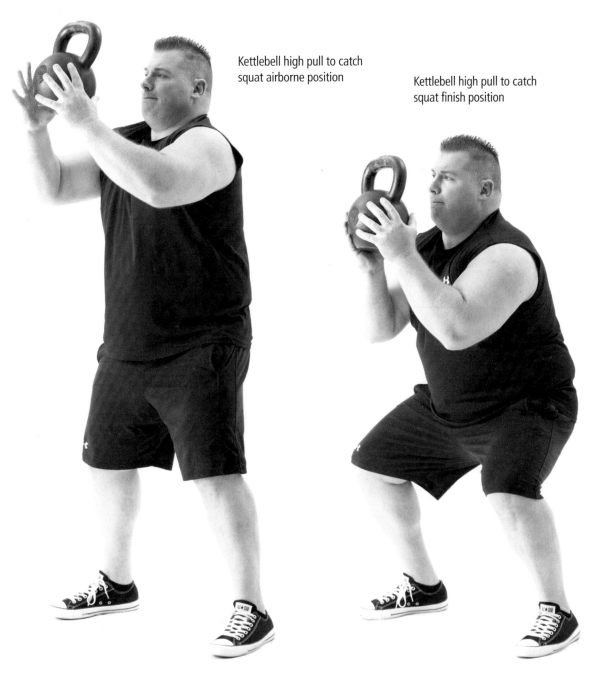

Kettlebell high pull to catch squat airborne position

Kettlebell high pull to catch squat finish position

# Single Kettlebell Walking Swing

Grasp a heavy kettlebell, and hike it between your legs while hinging at the hips. Explosively swing the kettlebell upward to chest level. As the kettlebell reaches the peak of the swing, step forward with your right foot followed by your left. The steps need to be quick, as you need to be set before the kettlebell can be swung backwards again through your legs.

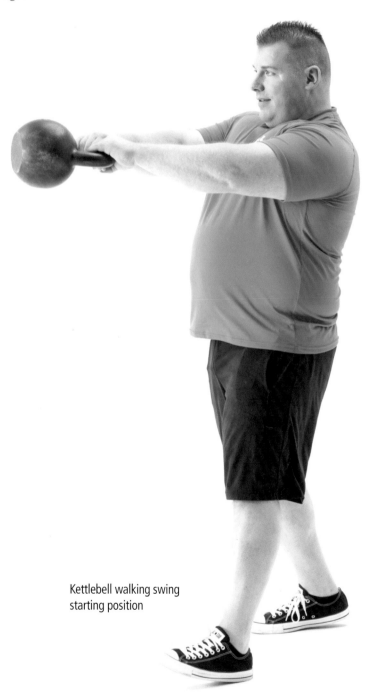

Kettlebell walking swing
starting position

Repeat this swinging movement, but this time step with the left foot first. Alternate the starting foot on every swing. Continue the exercise for the required time.

**Performance Point:** The timing of the step is very important, wait until the moment of weight-lessness of the swing before you step.

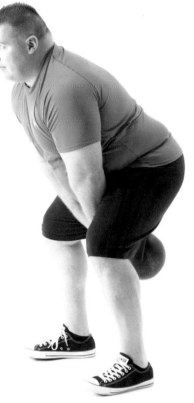

Kettlebell walking swing middle position

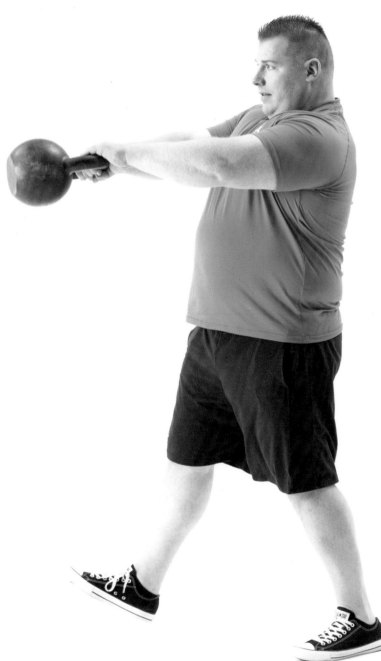

Kettlebell walking swing finish position

# Single Kettlebell Jump Squats

Pick up a kettlebell by its horns to chest level with elbows tight to the sides. Squat down and when you reach the bottom position, explosively jump up into the air. Your feet should come off the ground. Land softly, by allowing the balls of your feet to strike the ground first. Repeat the exercise for the time requirement.

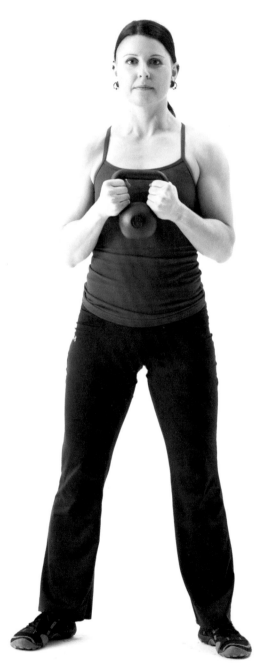

Single kettlebell jump squat starting position

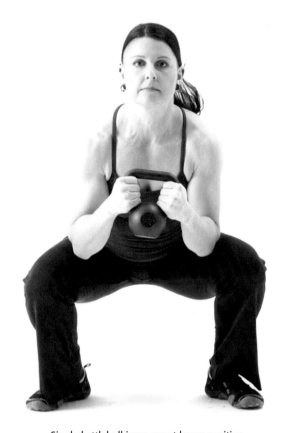

Single kettlebell jump squat lower position

**Performance Point:** Be sure to keep the kettlebell locked into position for the duration of this exercise. Don't allow the handle to hit you in the chin.

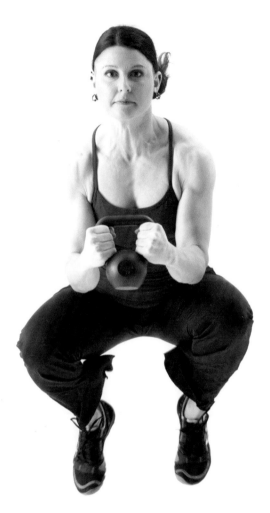

Single kettlebell jump squat airborne position

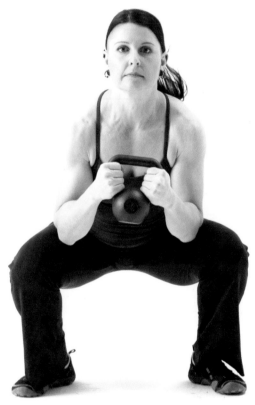

Single kettlebell jump squat finish position

## Double Kettlebell Jump Squats

Place a kettlebell on the outside of each your feet. Squat down and grasp the kettlebells. Rise to a standing position. Now, squat down without letting the kettlebells touch the floor. When you've reached this bottom position, explosively jump up into the air. As you become airborne, allow the elbows to flex slightly. You should land on the balls of your feet first, to help absorb the impact. Repeat the exercise until the time requirement is met.

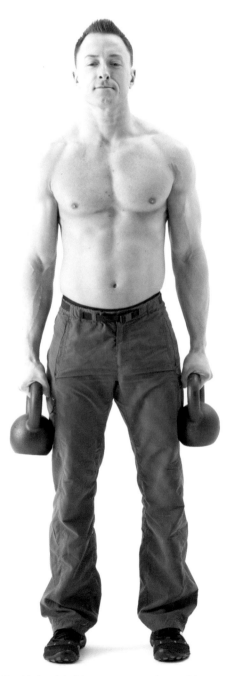

Double kettlebell jump squat starting position

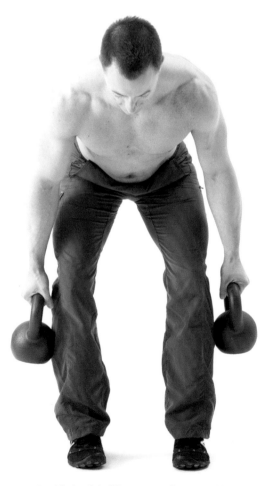

Double kettlebell jump squat lower position

70

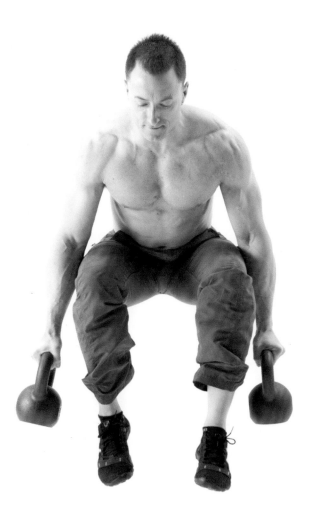

Double kettlebell jump squat airborne position

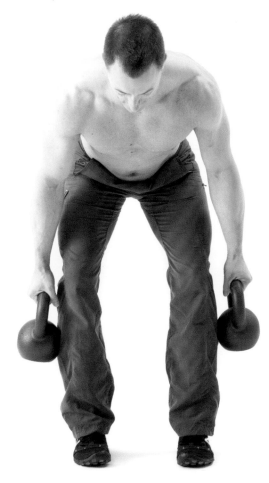

Double kettlebell jump squat finish position

# Double Kettlebell Calf Jumps

Begin with a kettlebell on the outside of each foot. Squat down and grasp the kettlebells and stand up. From this position, using the power of your calves, explosively jump up. Keep your knees slightly bent as you repeat this jumping motion. Make sure to land on the balls of your feet to maximize power and safety during this exercise. Repeat the movement for the required time.

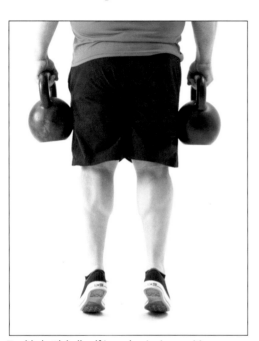

Double kettlebell calf jump beginning position

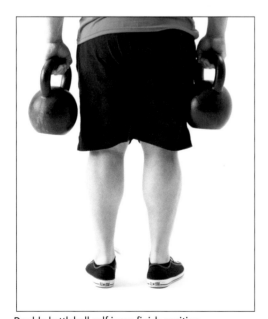

Double kettlebell calf jump finish position

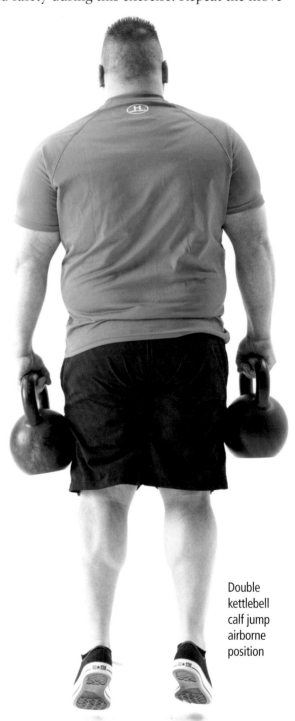

Double kettlebell calf jump airborne position

# Kettlebell Lateral Shuffle

Grasp the kettlebell by the horns and place it at chest level keeping the elbows tight to the body. Now, squat down until your thighs are slightly above parallel position to the ground. Pushing off your left foot began to shuffle your body to the right. After three or more repetitions, push off with your right foot and shuffle your body to the left. Change directions every 3 to 5 repetitions. Repeat the exercise for the required amount of time.

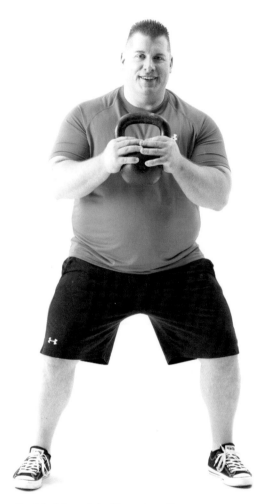

Kettlebell lateral shuffle start position

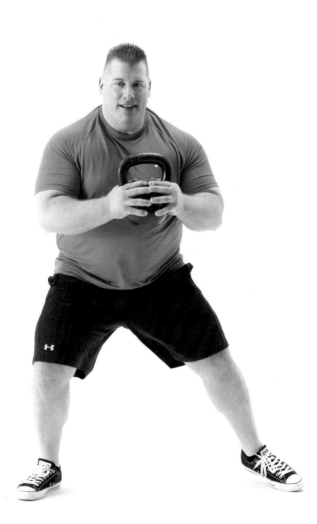

Kettlebell lateral shuffle shift position

**Performance Point:** It is essential to stay in the partial squat position for the duration of the exercise to maximize its benefits.

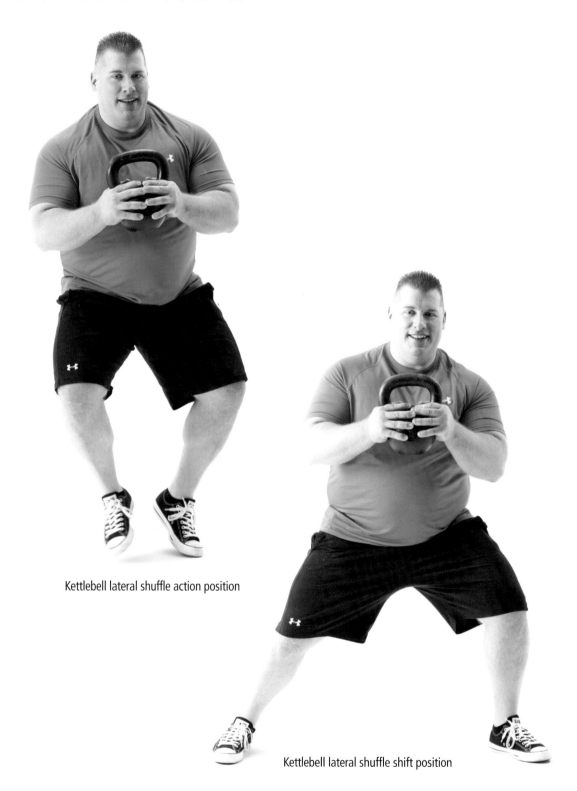

Kettlebell lateral shuffle action position

Kettlebell lateral shuffle shift position

## The Double Kettlebell Toe Curl

Begin by sitting on a bench allowing only your ankles to hang off the end. Place each of your feet through a light kettlebell. Now, curl your toes toward your kneecaps. Reverse the movement by pointing your toes away from your body. Repeat the exercise for the required amount of time.

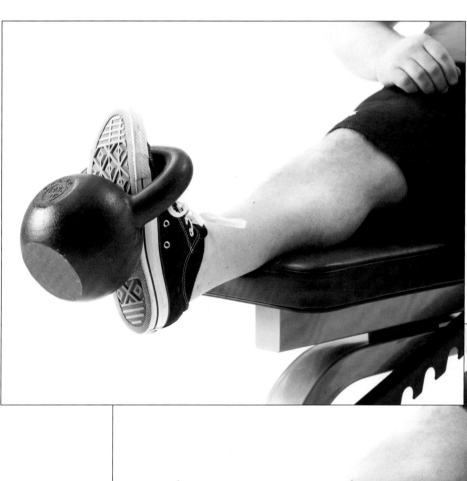

Double kettlebell toe curl finish position

Double kettlebell toe curl beginning position

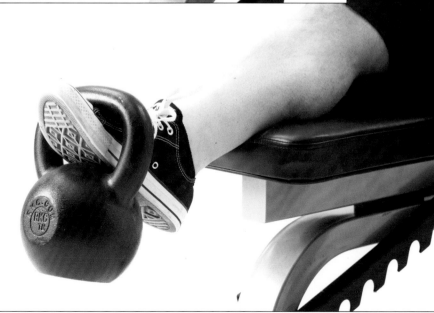

75

# Kettlebell Reverse Hyperextension

    To begin, find a table or bench that is higher than your hips. Facing the bench, place a light kettlebell in between your feet. Now, place your upper body from your waist up face down on the bench. Your hips should hinge on the end of the bench. Squeezing the kettlebell between your feet, explosively drive your heels backwards until your body is completely straight. Now, let the legs swing down to the starting position. Repeat this movement for the required time.

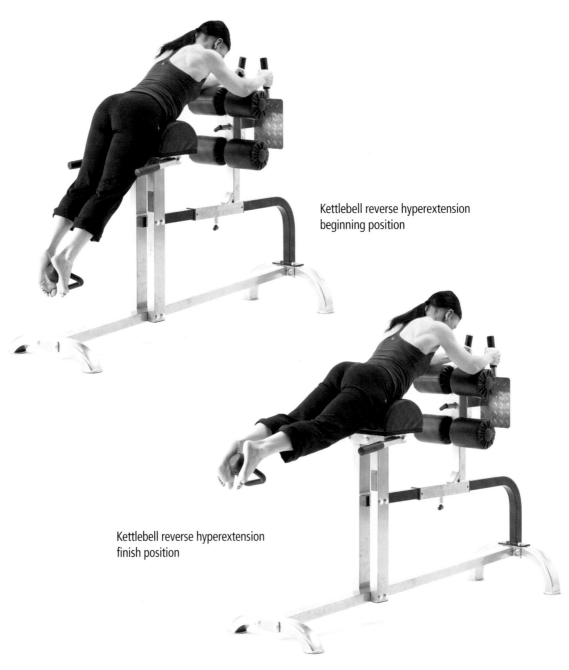

Kettlebell reverse hyperextension
beginning position

Kettlebell reverse hyperextension
finish position

# Kettlebell Dynamic Power Drills, Upper Body

### Double Kettlebell Rolling Speed Press

This is an excellent exercise to build upper body power. The rolling action of the exercise also increases mobility. To begin, lay on the floor with two kettlebells at your sides. Roll slightly to the right, and place your hand through the kettlebell handle. Now, roll slightly to your left and place your left hand through the kettlebell handle. You now should have the bells in the floor press position. Now punch up the right kettlebell while rolling toward your left side. Begin to actively pull down the right kettlebell as you punch the left kettlebell upward rolling toward your right. Continue this explosive punching in rolling action. You will find that there is a rhythmic nature to this exercise. Repeat the exercise for the required time.

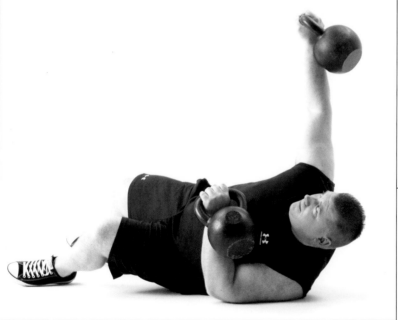

Double kettlebell
rolling speed press
right punch position

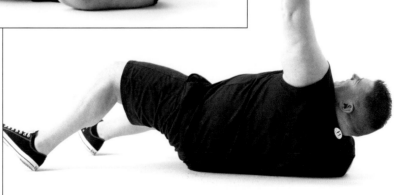

Double kettlebell
rolling speed press
left punch position

# Double Kettlebell Speed See Saw Press

Start by cleaning to kettlebells to the rack position. Explosively punch the right kettlebell straight up into the air. Now, actively begin to pull the right kettlebell down to the rack position while simultaneously punching the left kettlebell into the air. This movement should be performed as quickly as possible without compromising good technique. Continue the exercise for the required amount of time.

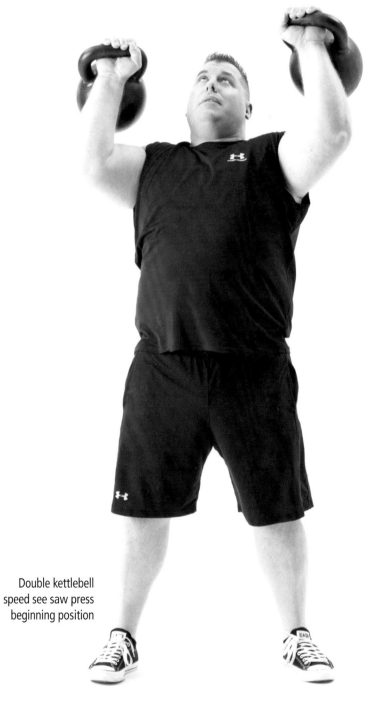

Double kettlebell
speed see saw press
beginning position

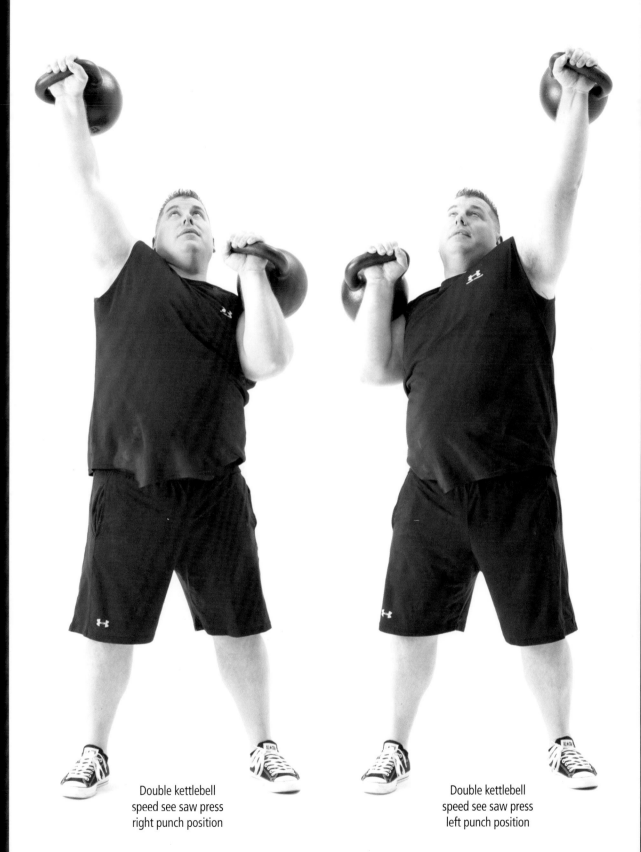

Double kettlebell
speed see saw press
right punch position

Double kettlebell
speed see saw press
left punch position

## Kettlebell High Pull From Squat

Even though this exercise involves the lower body, it is a great developer of the shoulders and traps. Begin by placing a kettlebell between your feet. Squat down and grasp the handle with both hands. Now, drive your feet through the floor as you pull the kettlebell straight up just below chin level. Really concentrate on squeezing your shoulder blades together and driving with the elbows during the pull.

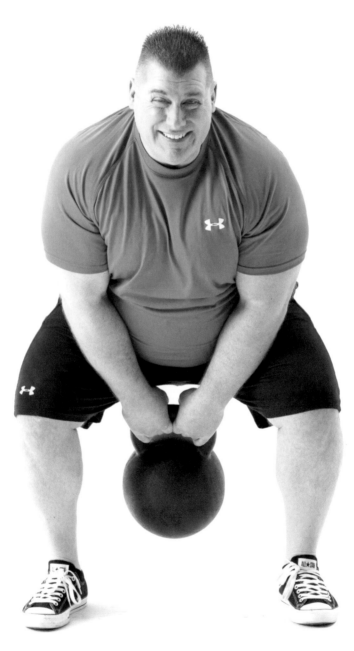

Kettlebell high pull from squat beginning position

Allow the bell to have a controlled fall towards the starting point of the exercise. Do not let the bell touch the ground. Repeat the pulling motion when the bell reaches 6 to 8 inches away from the ground. Repeat the exercise for the required amount of time.

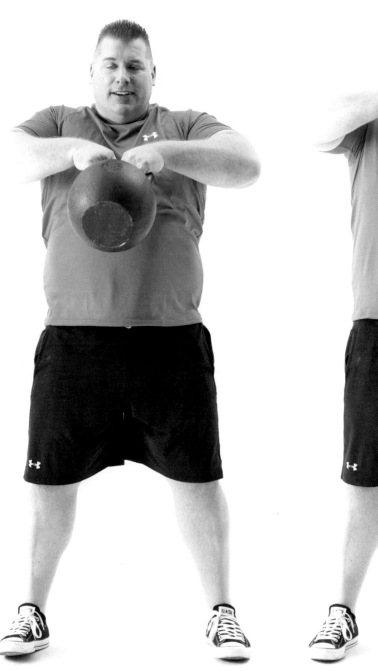

Kettlebell high pull from squat middle position

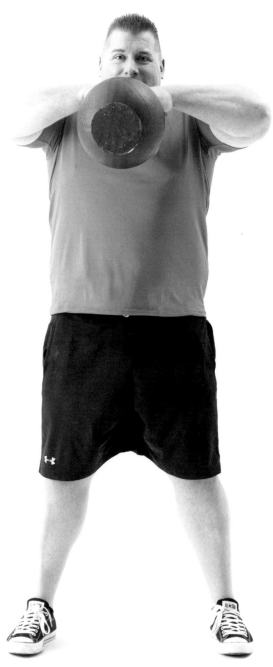

Kettlebell high pull from squat finish position

## Double Kettlebell Speed Row

Place a pair kettlebells on the insides of your feet. It is a good idea to perform this exercise on a rubber mat or outside. Keeping your back straight, hinged at the hips, lean forward and grasp the kettlebells. Using your lat muscles, explosively row the right kettlebell up while pushing the left kettlebell into the ground. Now, punch the right kettlebell down into the ground while explosively rowing the left kettlebell up. The punching motion teaches the body to absorb impact as a kettlebell hits the ground. This is an excellent exercise for increasing full body power. Repeat the exercise for the required amount of time.

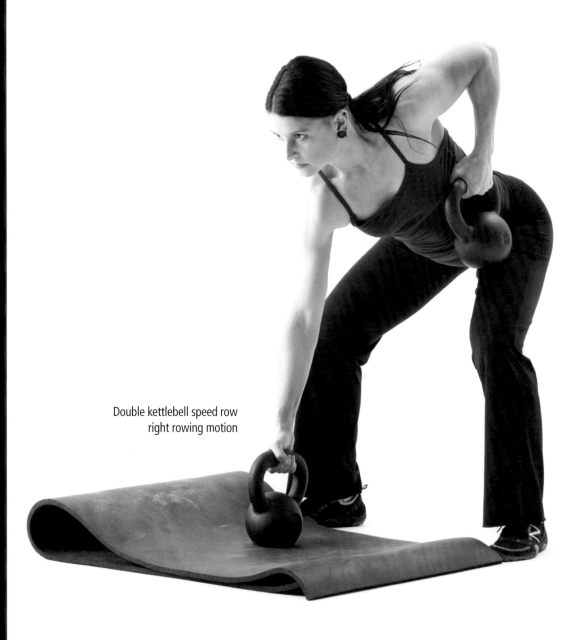

Double kettlebell speed row
right rowing motion

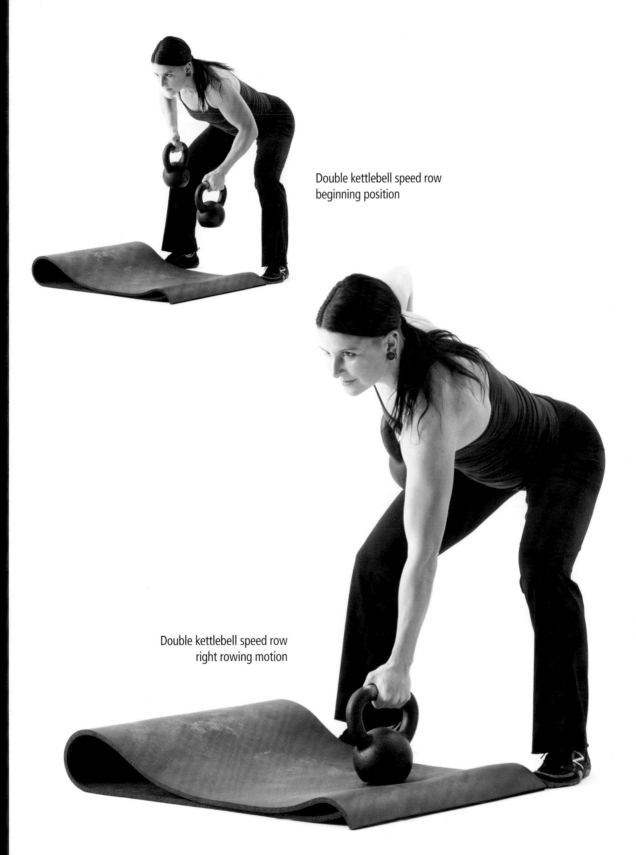

Double kettlebell speed row
beginning position

Double kettlebell speed row
right rowing motion

# Kettlebell Hand-To-Hand Swings

Start the exercise with a kettlebell sitting in between your feet. Grasp the kettlebell with one hand and while hinging at your hips, hike the bell back between your legs. Now, explosively drive with the hips and reverse the movement. As the kettlebell reaches the peak of the swing, let go of the kettlebell and catch it with the opposite hand.

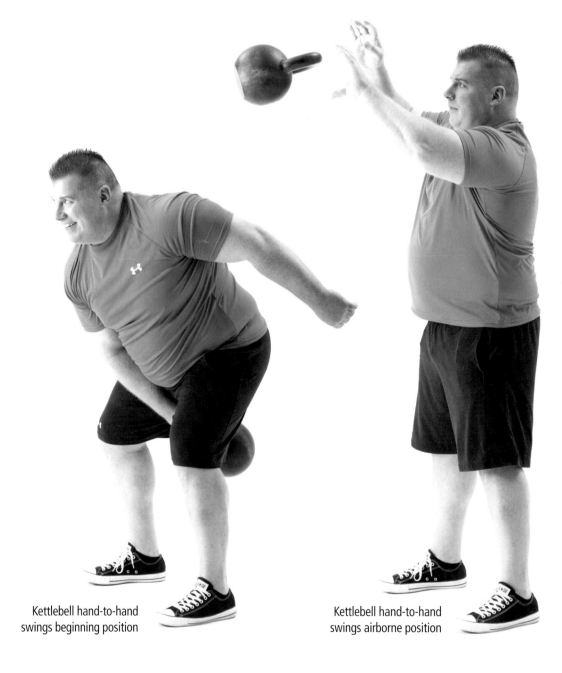

Kettlebell hand-to-hand
swings beginning position

Kettlebell hand-to-hand
swings airborne position

Allow the kettlebell to swing back between your legs and repeat the movement for the required amount of time. This exercise will develop your coordination, power, and grip.

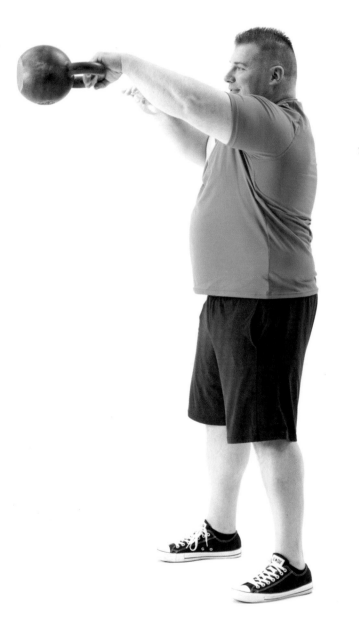

Kettlebell hand-to-hand
swings catch position

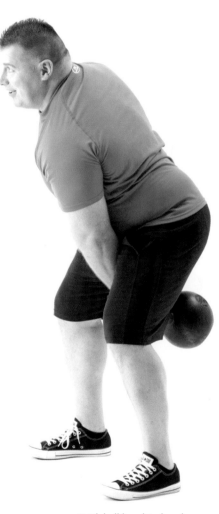

Kettlebell hand-to-hand
swings finish position

## Kettlebell Primal Shakers Standing Position

Kettlebell primal shaking is an exercise right out of the animal kingdom. We see the gorilla perform this basic movement as he shakes trees and other vegetation. The gorilla builds tremendous power by doing this. We will be performing primal shaking while holding a kettlebell.

Bring a kettlebell to chest level and crush it with your palms just below the horns. Begin to explosively push the kettlebell away from you and then immediately pull it back toward you. Do not let your elbows become fully extended during the exercise.

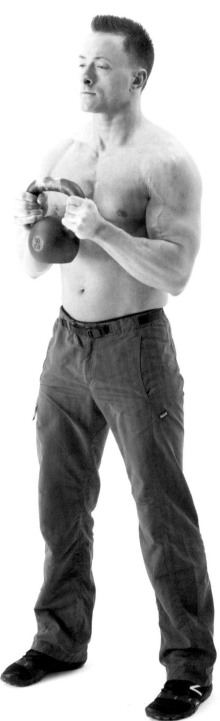

Kettlebell primal shakers
standing beginning position

The movement should be performed as fast as you can go while maintaining control. Continue this shaking motion for the required amount of time.

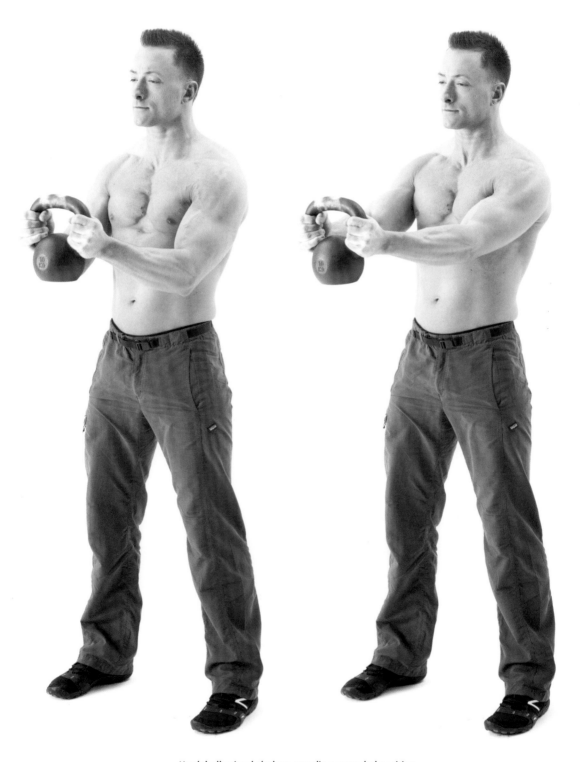

Kettlebell primal shakers standing extended position

# Kettlebell Primal Shakers Sit-Up Position

For this exercise you will need to have your legs locked in the midrange sit-up position. You may use a partner or a barbell to assist you in this exercise. Begin by sitting down and placing your feet under a barbell. Bring a kettlebell to chest level and crush it with your palms just below the horns. Tighten your core and lean back into the midrange portion of a sit-up. Now, begin to explosively shake the kettlebell by using short pushing and pulling movements. Do not let your elbows become fully extended during the exercise. The movement should be as fast as you can go while maintaining control. Continue this shaking motion for the required amount of time.

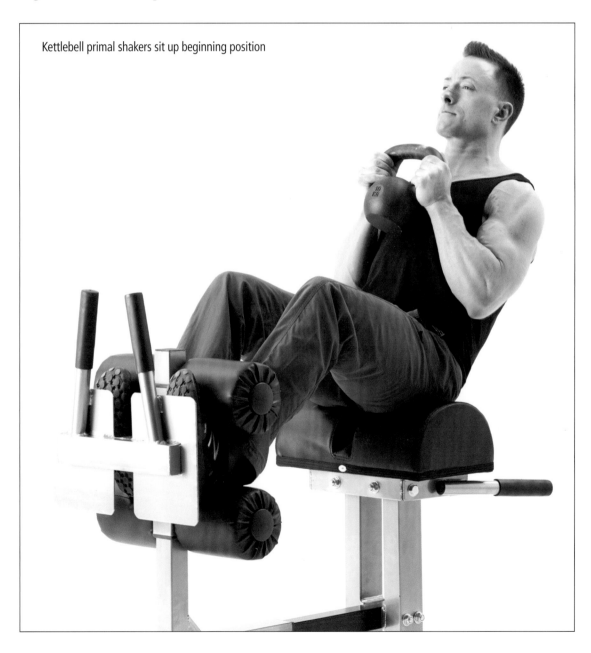

Kettlebell primal shakers sit up beginning position

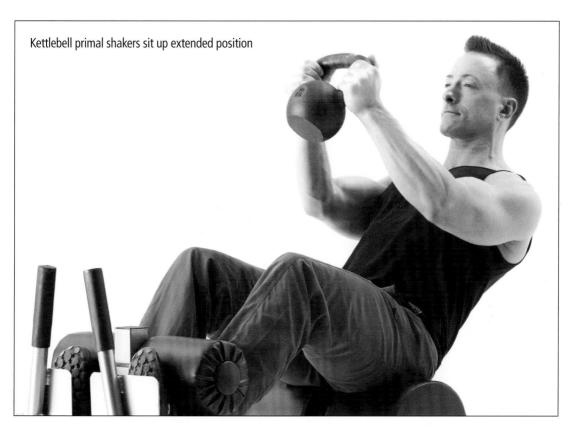

Kettlebell primal shakers sit up extended position

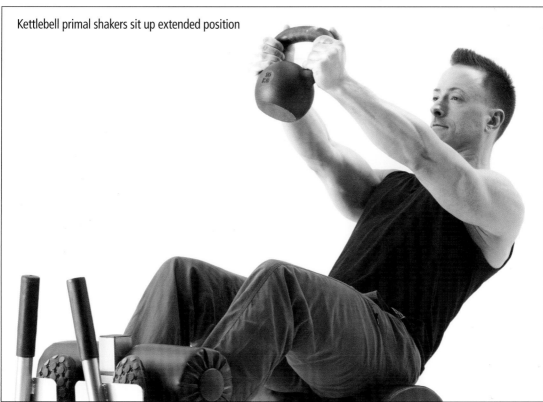

Kettlebell primal shakers sit up extended position

## Kettlebell Front Raise Snatch

I first saw this kettlebell exercise performed by John Brookfield. The kettlebell front raise snatch builds power and mass into the shoulders. The beginning form is like the old school swing snatch. Keeping your arm straight, begin to snatch the kettlebell. When the kettlebell nears chest level, allow the bell to flip over to the top of your wrist. This is accomplished by punching the bell forward. Once you are in the top position, pause for a moment before flipping the kettlebell over and swinging to the start position. The pause places tremendous stress on the shoulders. Repeat this movement for the required time.

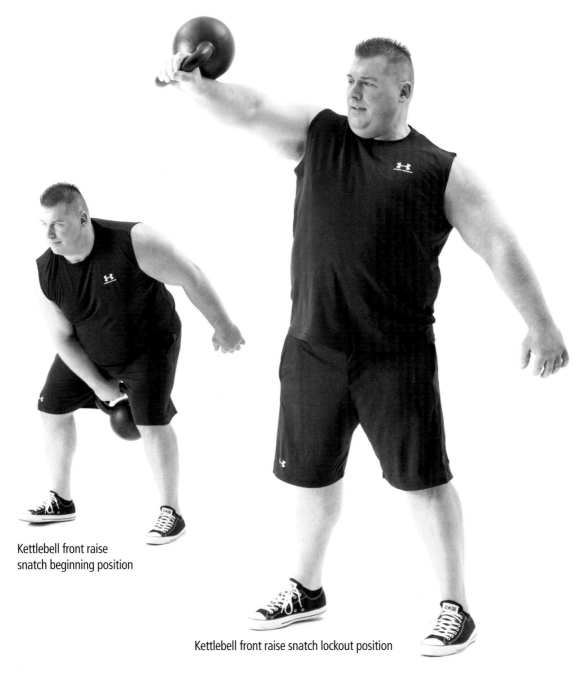

Kettlebell front raise
snatch beginning position

Kettlebell front raise snatch lockout position

# Double Kettlebell Hang Cleans

Pick up two kettlebells so that you are in the standing position. Driving your feet through the floor, explosively pull the kettlebells into the rack position.

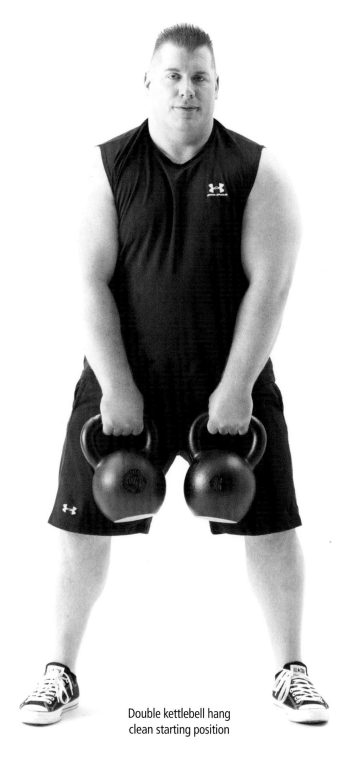

Double kettlebell hang
clean starting position

Brace your core so that you can absorb the impact. Push the bells off of the racked position and catch them in the hang position. Repeat the exercise for the required amount of time.

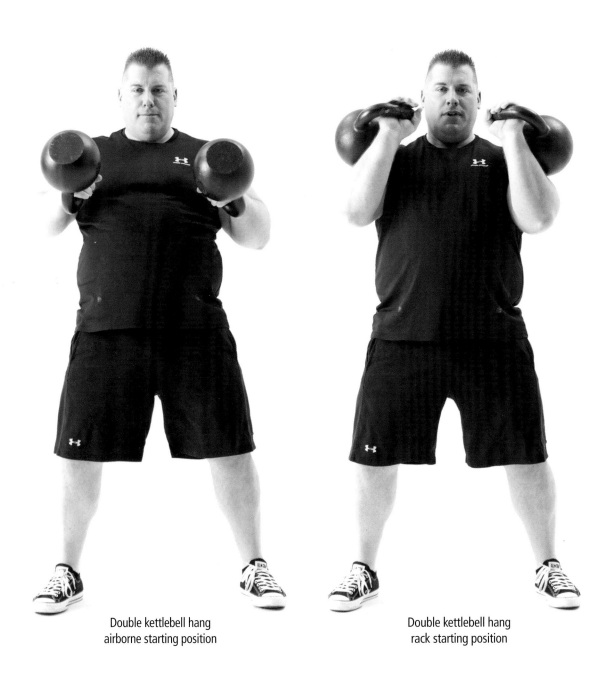

Double kettlebell hang
airborne starting position

Double kettlebell hang
rack starting position

# The Double Kettlebell Bear Crawl

Begin by placing a pair of kettlebells in front of you.   Squat down and grasp the kettlebells and step back with your feet so that you are in a modified plank position. Your glutes should be higher than a standard plank. Now, lift and move the right kettlebell forward while simultaneously stepping your left foot forward. Repeat the movement with the left kettlebell on the right foot.  Repeat the crawling movement for the required time.

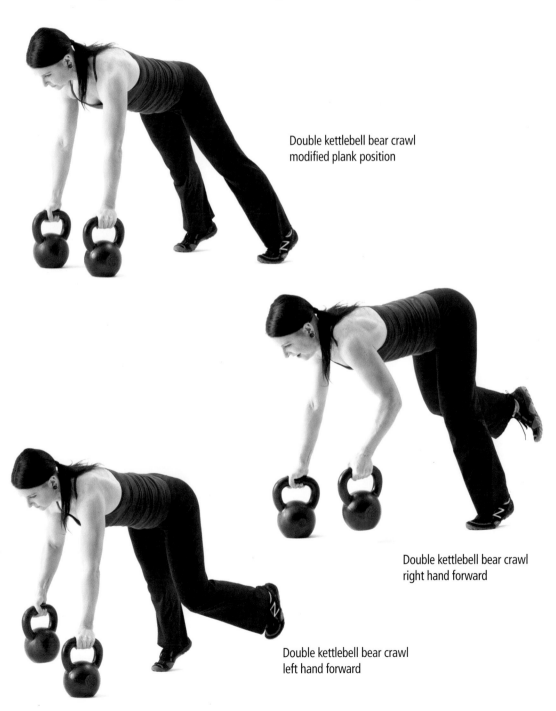

Double kettlebell bear crawl
modified plank position

Double kettlebell bear crawl
right hand forward

Double kettlebell bear crawl
left hand forward

# The Kettlebell Cross Body Snatch

Start by placing the kettlebell touching the inside of your right foot. Grasp the handle with your left hand and snatch the kettlebell in one powerful motion across your body to the top lockout position. Bring the kettlebell to the rack position and then lower it to the inside of your left foot. Now perform the snatch with the right hand.

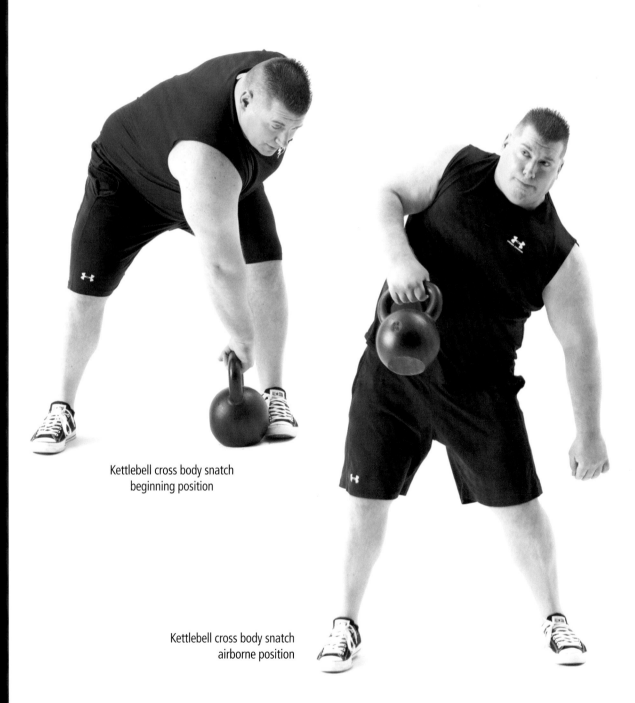

Kettlebell cross body snatch
beginning position

Kettlebell cross body snatch
airborne position

Alternate sides after every repetition. This exercise builds tremendous power in the core and taxes all the stabilizer muscles. Repeat this exercise for the required time.

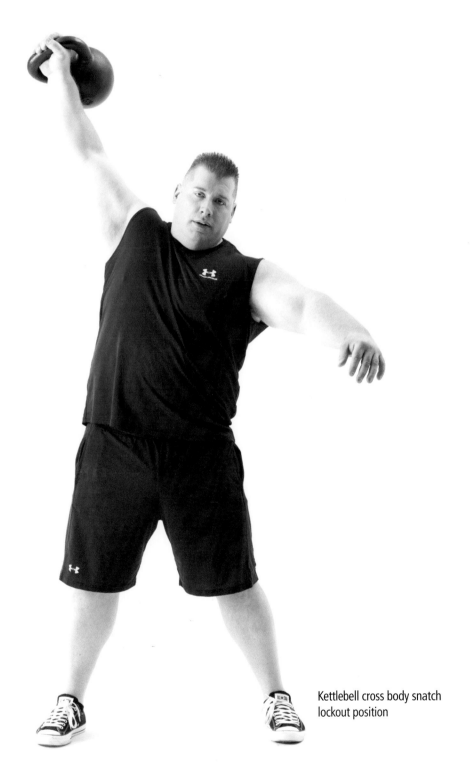

Kettlebell cross body snatch lockout position

# The Kettlebell Seated Twist

From a seated position grasp the kettlebell by the horns and place it at chest level. Now, pressurize your core and lean back bringing your bent legs off the ground. Your glutes should be the only thing touching the floor. Rotate your upper body slowly to the right and then slowly to the left. Repeat this exercise for the required amount of time.

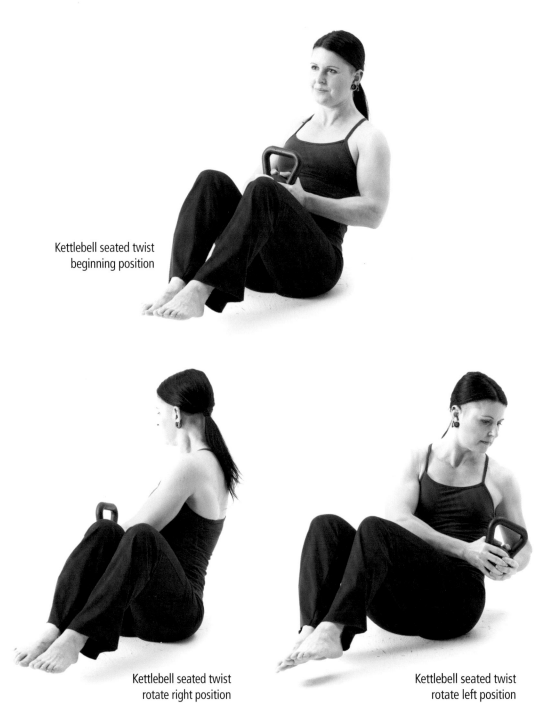

Kettlebell seated twist
beginning position

Kettlebell seated twist
rotate right position

Kettlebell seated twist
rotate left position

# Kettlebell Isometrics Lower Body

## The Double Kettlebell Isometric Wall Squat Quadriceps Emphasis

Clean a pair of kettlebells to the rack position while standing near a wall. Now, squat down until your thighs are parallel with the ground and your back is flat against the wall. Using your feet try to push your back through the wall. Gradually increase tension and squeeze the quads while you power exhale through the mouth. Continue this isometric contraction for 7 to 12 seconds.

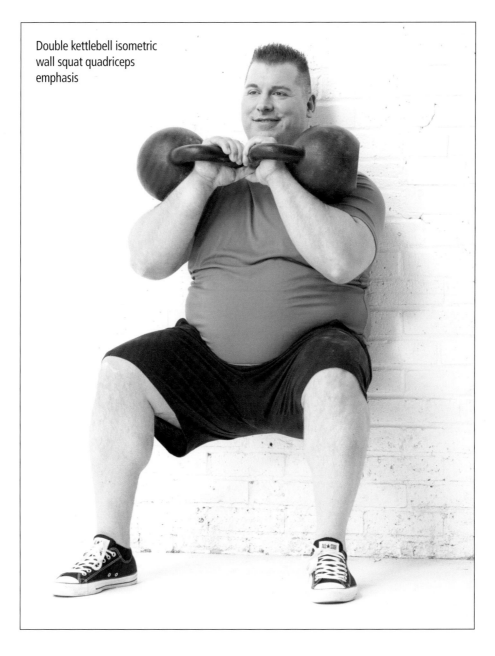

Double kettlebell isometric wall squat quadriceps emphasis

# The Double Kettlebell Isometric Wall Squat Hamstring Emphasis

Clean a pair of kettlebells to the rack position while standing near a wall. Now, squat down until your thighs are parallel with the ground and your back is flat against the wall. Now, drive your heels into the floor trying to pull them into the wall. Gradually increase tension and squeeze the hamstrings while you power exhale through the mouth. Continue this isometric contraction for 7 to 12 seconds.

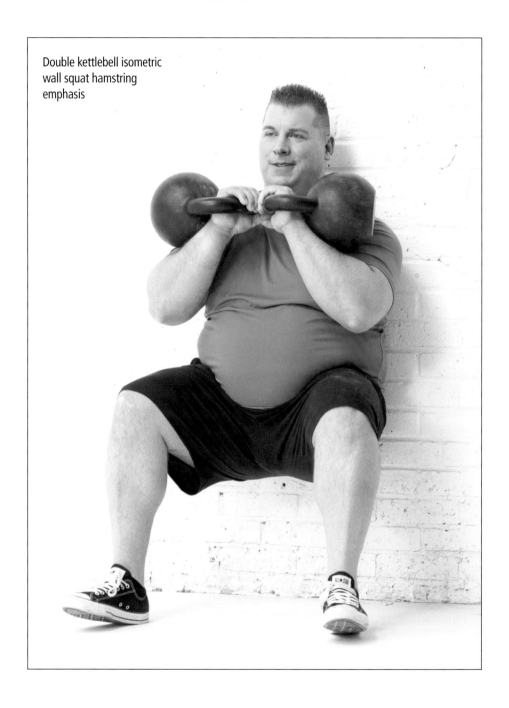

Double kettlebell isometric wall squat hamstring emphasis

## The Double Kettlebell Spread The Floor Isometric Squat

Take two heavy kettlebells and turn them on their sides allowing the bottoms of the bells to touch the outside of your feet. Now squat down until your thighs are parallel with the floor. Now, try to spread the floor with your feet as you place pressure against the kettlebells. Gradually increase tension and squeeze the muscles in your legs as you power exhale through the mouth. Continue this isometric contraction for 7 to 12 seconds.

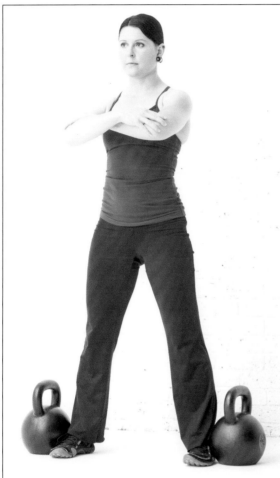

Double kettlebell spread the floor
isometric squat top position

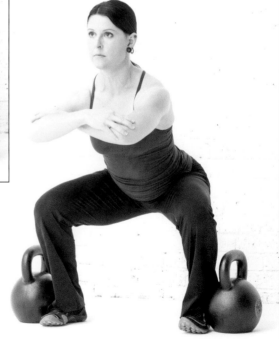

Double kettlebell spread the floor
isometric squat bottom position

# The Kettlebell Hyperextension Isometric Contraction

Position yourself on a hyperextension bench while holding a kettlebell by the horns tight to your chest. Perform the hyperextension exercise stopping in the top position. Squeeze and contract your lower back while holding in this position. Power exhale through the mouth as you continue this isometric contraction for 7 to 12 seconds.

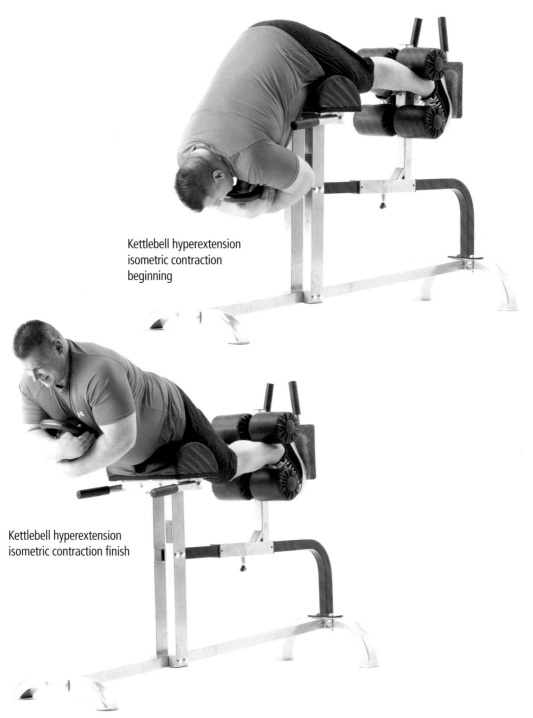

Kettlebell hyperextension
isometric contraction
beginning

Kettlebell hyperextension
isometric contraction finish

# The Double Kettlebell Calf Raise Isometric Contraction

Grasp a pair of kettlebells and hold them at your sides. Now, raise your heels off of the ground and squeeze your calf muscles hard. Power exhale through the mouth, as you continue this isometric contraction for 7 to 12 seconds.

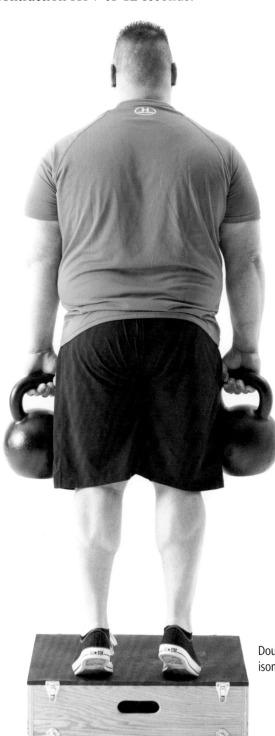

Double kettlebell calf raise
isometric contraction

# Kettlebell Isometrics Upper Body

## The Kettlebell Chest Crush Isometric

Hold a kettlebell at chest height gripping it with the palms just below the horns. With your elbows flared out to your sides, begin to apply tension by trying to crush the kettlebell. Squeeze and contract your chest muscles for the duration of the exercise. Power exhale to the mouth, as you continue this isometric contraction for 7 to 12 seconds.

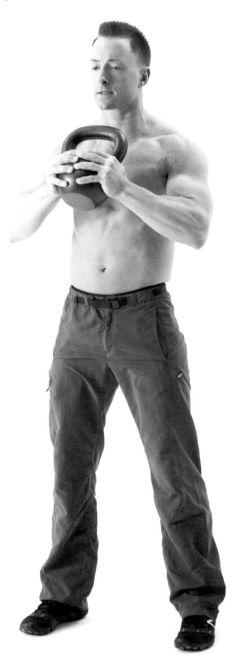

Kettlebell chest crush
isometric

# The Upside Down Kettlebell Chest Crush In Plank Position

Place a kettlebell on the floor so that the handle is upside down. Using your palms crush the kettlebell, and step your feet back into the plank position. Lower your upper body until it is just above the bell. Continue to apply tension as you squeeze the chest and try to crush the bell. Power exhale to the mouth as you continue this isometric contraction for 7 to 12 seconds.

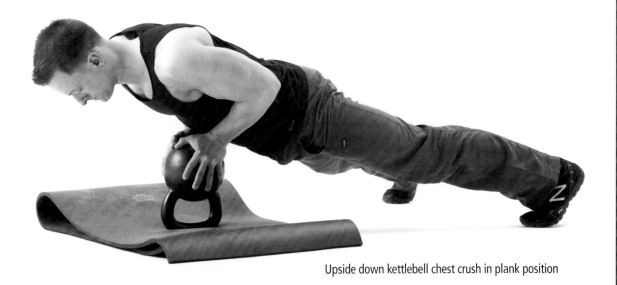

Upside down kettlebell chest crush in plank position

# The Double Kettlebell Isometric Lateral Raise

Pick up a pair of heavy kettlebells and hold them in your sides. Now, try to perform a lateral shoulder raise. Squeeze the shoulders hard as you try to raise the bells. The feeling is similar to that of standing in a doorway raising your arms against it. Continue to apply tension throughout the duration of the exercise. Power exhale to the mouth as you continue this isometric contraction for 7 to 12 seconds.

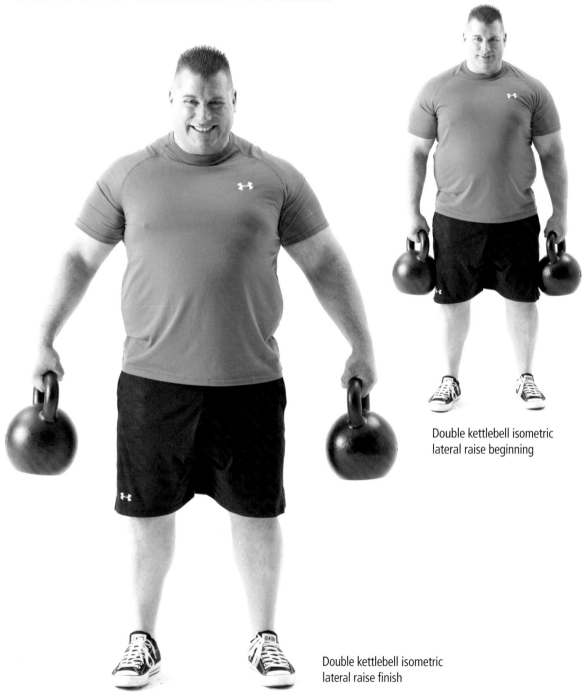

Double kettlebell isometric
lateral raise beginning

Double kettlebell isometric
lateral raise finish

# The Kettlebell Isometric Chest Pull

Even though this exercise is called a chest pull, it really targets the upper back muscles. To begin, raise a kettlebell to chest level by grasping the horns. Now, with your elbows flared, try to pull the handle apart. Squeeze the shoulder blades together as you continue to apply tension by pulling the kettlebell handle. Power exhale through the mouth as you continue this isometric contraction for 7 to 12 seconds.

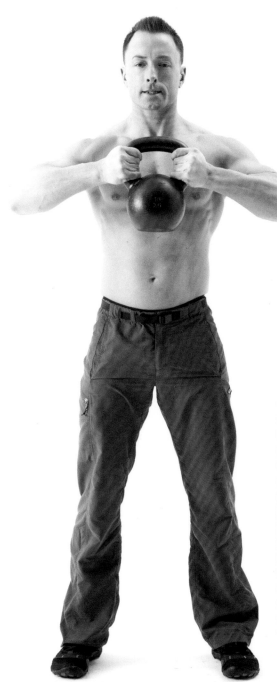

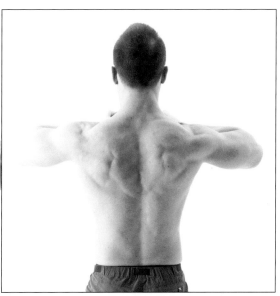

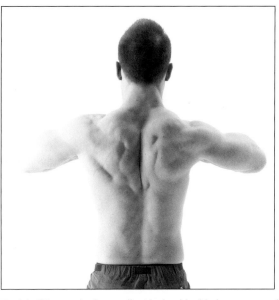

Kettlebell isometric chest pull with shoulder blades contracted

## The Kettlebell Isometric Shoulder Press

There are several options in performing this exercise. The goal is to create a weight that is too heavy for you to press.

Option 1. Choose a heavy kettlebell that you can clean, but are not able to press.

Option 2.  You can attach a nylon belt or daisy chain to the kettlebell handle and attach it to a weighted object on the floor.

Option 3.  You can stack two kettlebells on top of each other.

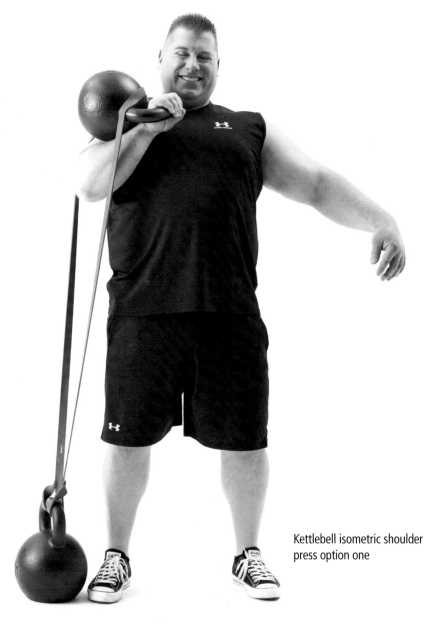

Kettlebell isometric shoulder press option one

Once you have chosen your press option, clean the kettlebell to the rack position. Now, create tension as you try to press the kettlebell upward. Make sure to squeeze the lats and shoulders throughout the duration of the exercise. Power exhale through the mouth as you continue this isometric contraction for 7 to 12 seconds.

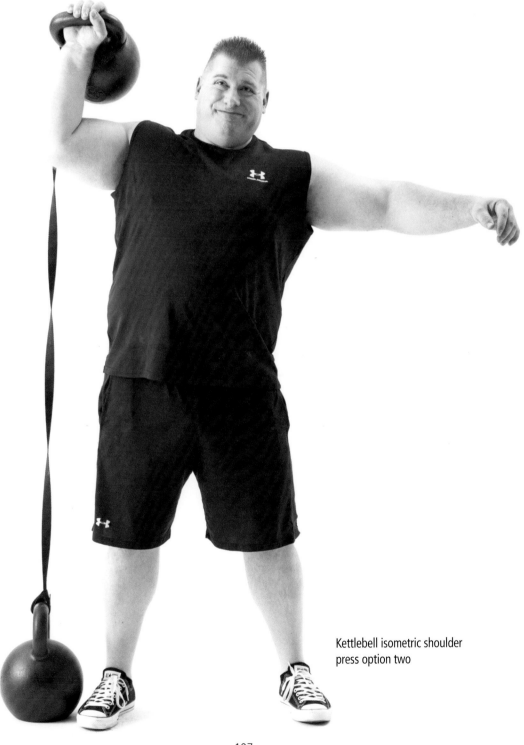

Kettlebell isometric shoulder
press option two

# The Double Kettlebell Isometric Row

Position two heavy kettlebells just outside of your feet. Hinging at the hips and keeping your back straight, sit backwards until your hands can reach the bells. Inhale, crush the handles, and row the bells to the top position. Hold this position as you create an intense contraction in your upper back. Try to squeeze your shoulder blades together. Power exhale through the mouth as you continue this isometric contraction for 7 to 12 seconds.

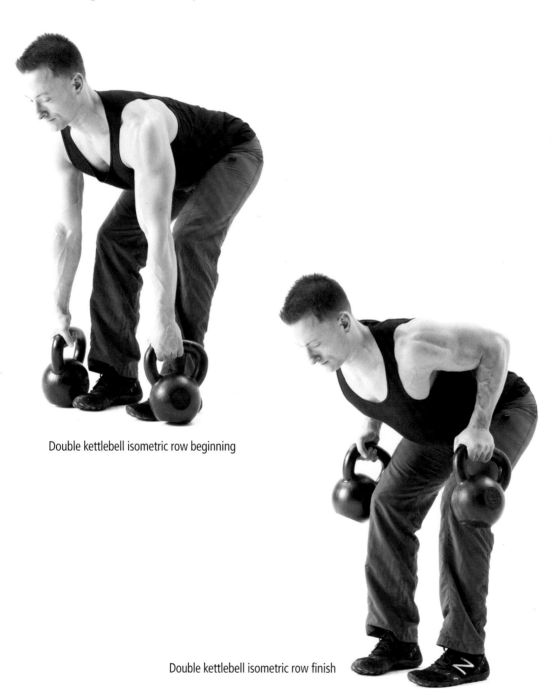

Double kettlebell isometric row beginning

Double kettlebell isometric row finish

## The Kettlebell Isometric Pull-Up

Hang a heavy kettlebell around your waist with a dipping belt. Grab the pull-up bar with an overhand grip. Now, try to pull yourself up. Create tension by squeezing the lats throughout the duration of the exercise. Power exhale through the mouth as you continue this isometric contraction for 7 to 12 seconds.

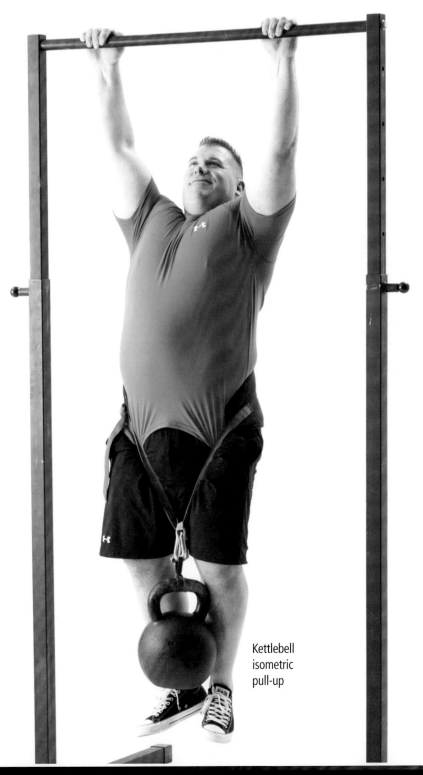

Kettlebell
isometric
pull-up

# Kettlebell Isometric Crunch

To begin, lay down on your back with your knees bent. Grasp the kettlebell by the horns with both hands and lock it out straight over your chest. Keeping your lower back on the floor, slowly crunch up and create an intense abdominal contraction. Hold this position for the duration of the exercise. Power exhale through the mouth as you continue this isometric contraction for 7 to 12 seconds.

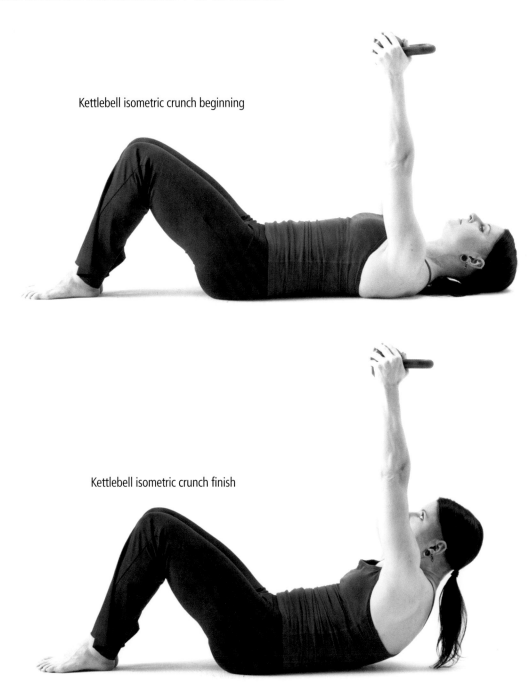

Kettlebell isometric crunch beginning

Kettlebell isometric crunch finish

# The Kettlebell Towel Crush

Wrap a small towel around the handle of a heavy kettlebell. Pick the kettlebell up with one hand and stand up. Now, squeeze the towel and handle as hard as possible for 7 to 12 seconds. Set the kettlebell down and repeat the exercise with the other hand.

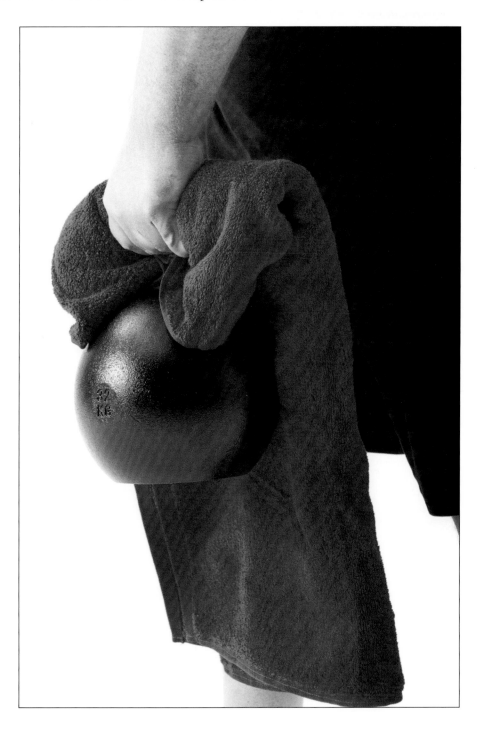

# Bodyweight Grinds Lower Body

### Regular Squats

Place your feet at shoulder width apart. Your toes should be slightly pointed outward. Now, slowly squat down and actively pull yourself into the bottom position. Keeping your chest high, drive your feet into the ground and squeeze the glutes as you rise to the starting position. Repeat this exercise for the required amount of repetitions.

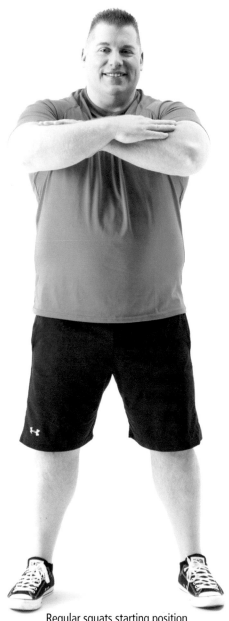

Regular squats starting position

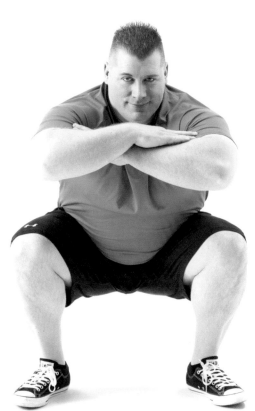

Regular squats finish position

## Ballet Squats

Begin by bringing your heels together with your toes pointing out at a 45° angle. Keeping your back straight, begin to squat down to the bottom position. Your heels should come off of the floor as you lower the body. Tense the glutes hard as you rise to the starting position. Repeat this exercise for the required amount of repetitions. Bodyweight ballet squats will create increased flexibility and balance when performed regularly.

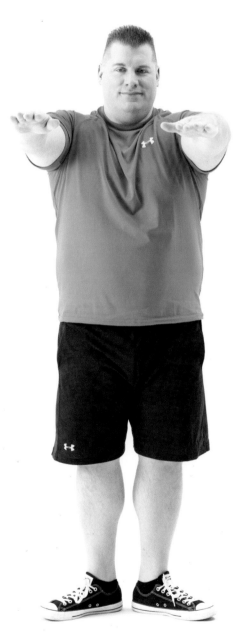

Ballet squats starting position

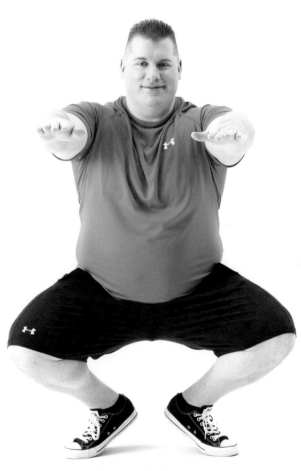

Ballet squats finish position

**Performance Point:** You may hold both arms out to the side if you are having trouble with balance.

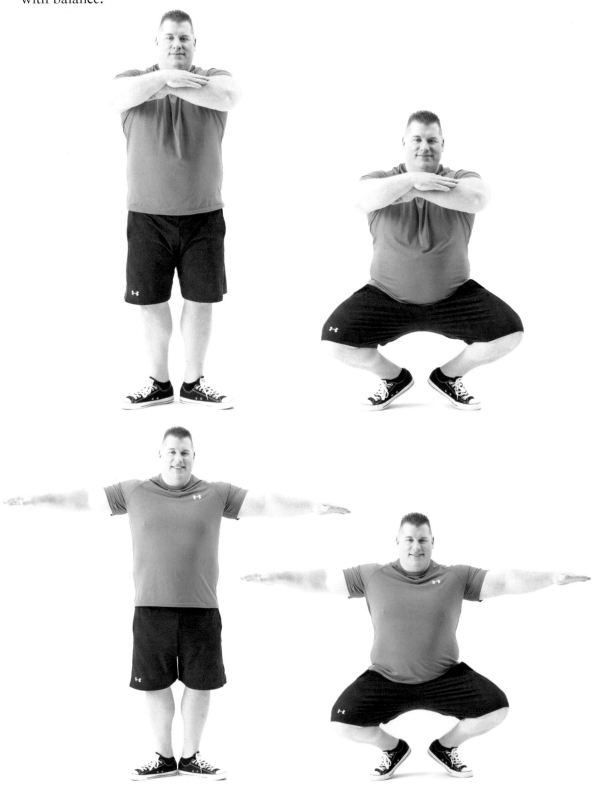

# The Front Elevation Lunge

To perform this exercise you will need a step that is six to ten inches in height. The front foot will be placed on the step increasing the range of motion, stretch, and muscle recruitment. Place the step two or more feet in front of your body. Step forward so that one foot is resting on the platform. The front foot should be in complete contact with the step. The rear heel will be off the floor. The front knee is partially bent. Lower the body toward the floor. To ascend, push hard with the elevated foot driving back up to the starting position.

**Performance Point:** Make sure to keep the back straight during this exercise. Fight the urge to lean forward. Finish all the repetitions on one leg before switching to the other leg.

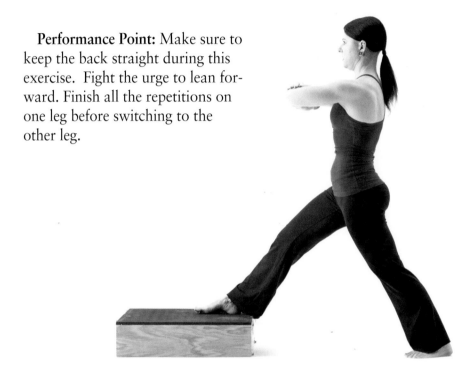

Front elevation lunge
beginning position

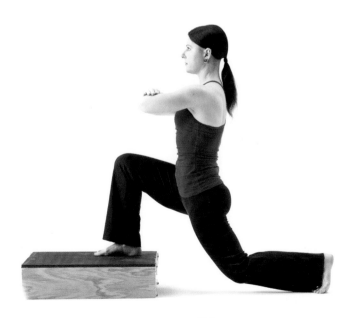

Front elevation lunge
finish position

# The Rear Elevation Lunge

Just as in the previous exercise, you will need a step or platform six to ten inches in height. This exercise really targets the quads. Place the step behind you. Lift one foot behind you until it is in contact with the top of the step. The heel of the elevated foot should not be touching the step. Pushing off with the rear foot, step the front foot forward. The knee of the front leg should be partially bent. This is the beginning position of the exercise.

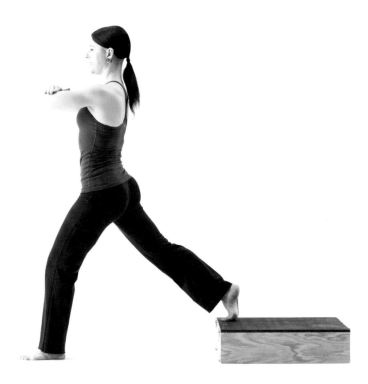

Rear elevation lunge
beginning position

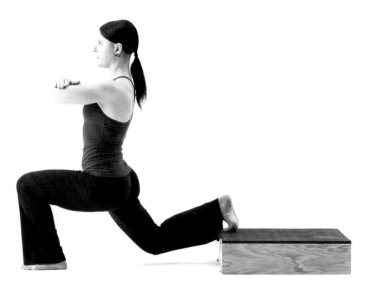

Rear elevation lunge
finish position

# Wide Squats

To begin, set your feet so that they are wider than shoulder width apart. Your toes should be slightly pointed outward. Actively pull yourself into the bottom position of the squat. Pause for a moment, then squeeze the glutes hard, as you drive up into the starting position. Repeat for the required amount of repetitions.

**Performance Point:** Performing wide squats on a regular basis will increase the health and flexibility of the hips.

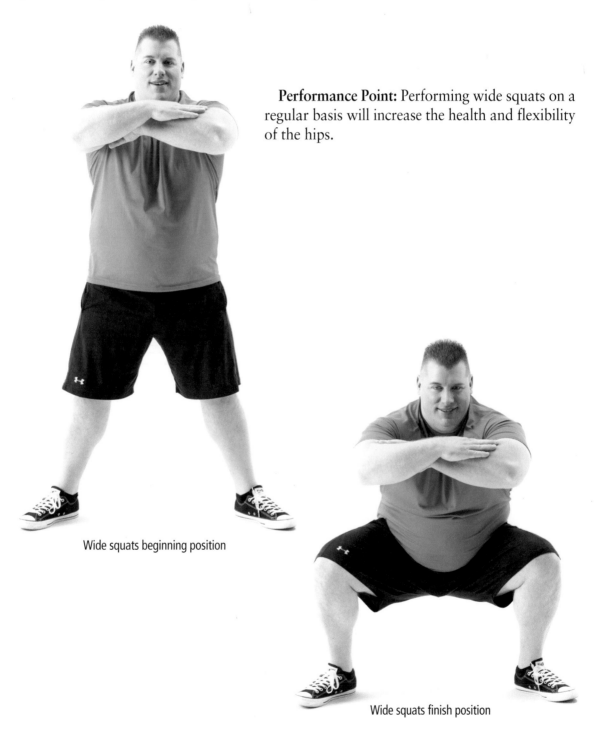

Wide squats beginning position

Wide squats finish position

## The Lateral Step Squat

Lateral movement is an essential skill used in competitive athletics. The lateral step squat also encourages hip mobility, body awareness, and balance.

Start by placing the feet slightly less than shoulder width apart. Raise the right foot six inches in the air while simultaneously pushing laterally with the left foot. Absorb the impact with the right foot as you pull yourself down into the squat position. Now, with chest high, and tensed glutes, drive upwards and laterally by pushing off of the right foot. The right foot will come off the ground again around six inches as you are returning to the starting position. Remember to power breathe to keep tension on the core. Now, repeat the movement in the opposite direction. Alternate sides until you complete the required amount of repetitions. This exercise takes some time to master.

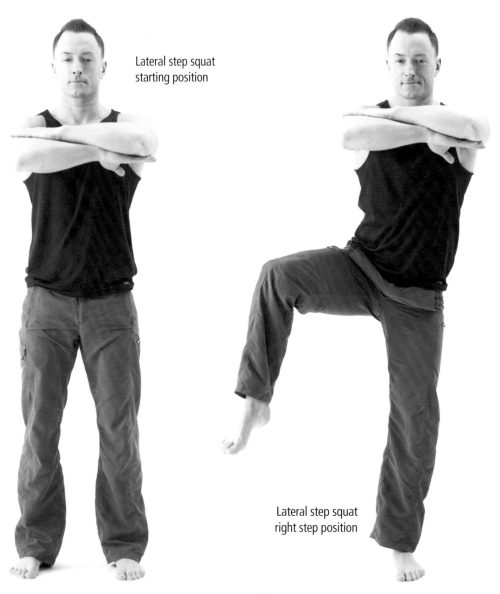

Lateral step squat
starting position

Lateral step squat
right step position

**Performance Point:** When moving laterally to the right, make sure that the left foot stays planted. When moving laterally to the left, the right foot should stay planted.

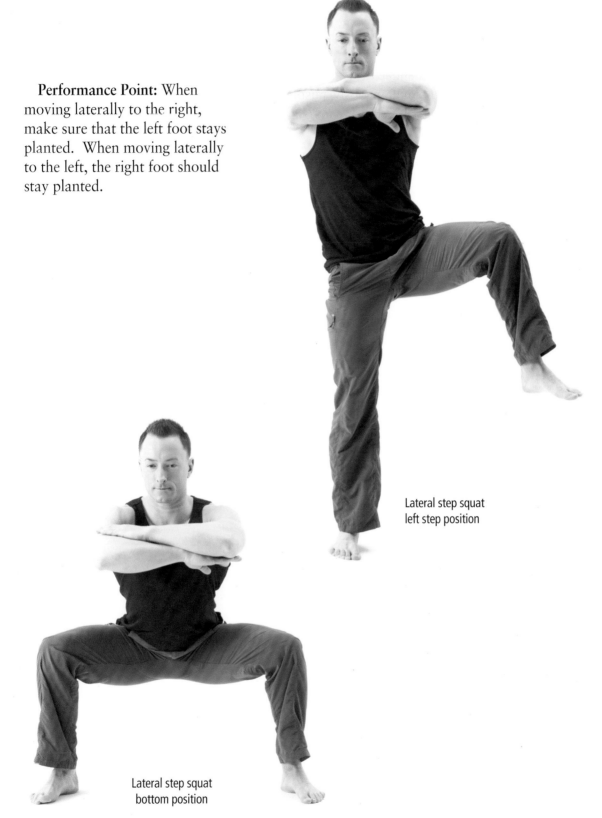

Lateral step squat
left step position

Lateral step squat
bottom position

# The Romanian Deadlift

To begin, please your feet about 8 to 12 inches apart. Now, interlock both hands behind your back. With your knees slightly bent, hinge at the hips and begin to bend forward. Continue to come forward until you feel a stretch in your hamstring muscles. Keeping your back straight return to the starting position. Repeat for the required amount of repetitions.

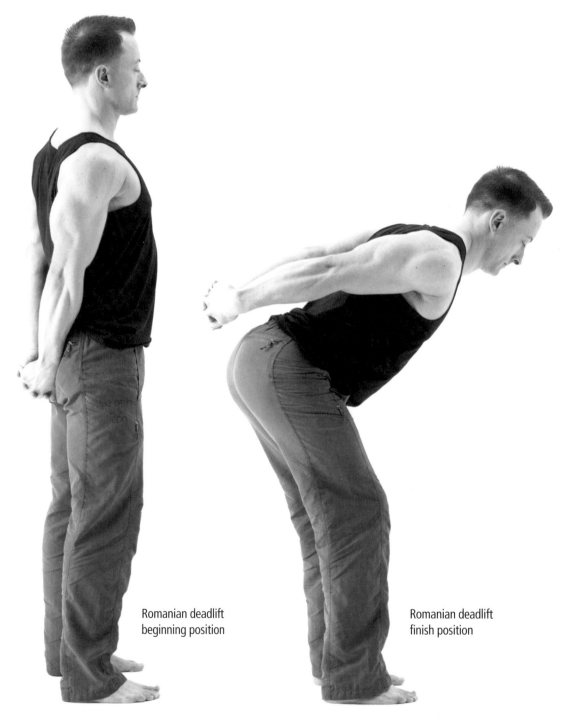

Romanian deadlift
beginning position

Romanian deadlift
finish position

# The Single Leg Deadlift

Start by placing your feet about 8 to 12 inches apart. Firmly plant your left foot on the ground and allow your knees to be slightly bent. Hinge at the hips and lean forward while simultaneously allowing the right leg to rise up straight behind you. The upper body and leg should move together. Return to the starting position. Complete all of the required repetitions on one leg before switching to the other leg.

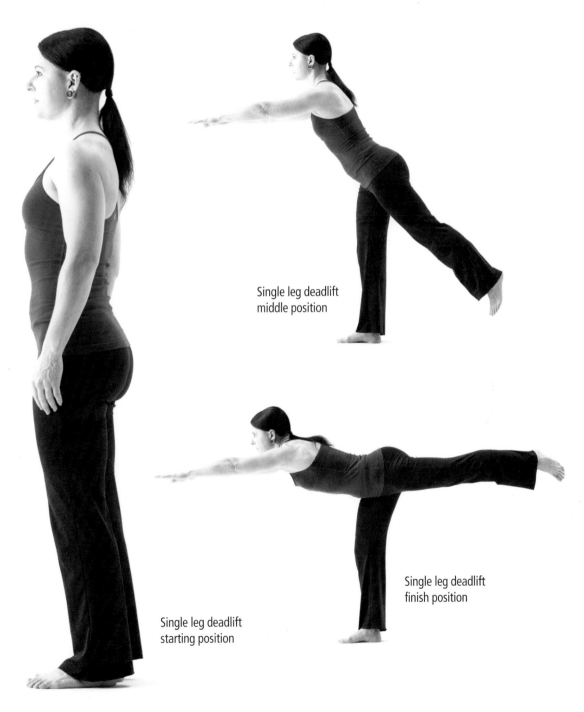

Single leg deadlift middle position

Single leg deadlift finish position

Single leg deadlift starting position

# The Glute Ham Raise

To perform this exercise, place your knees on a heavily padded surface. A folded over heavy-duty exercise mat works well for this purpose. Now, have a partner hold down your ankles or use a padded bar to anchor them. Inhale, squeeze your glutes and create tension in your posterior chain as you slowly lower your body to the floor bending only at the knees. Pause for a moment, inhale and reverse the movement. Place your hands in front of you to catch yourself in case you lose control. You not want to do a face plant. If you are having trouble with this exercise, you can perform the assisted glute ham raise. This is accomplished by pushing off with your hands in the lowered position. Repeat the exercise for the required amount of repetitions.

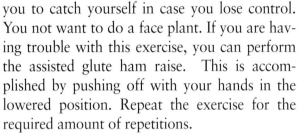
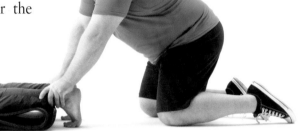

Glute ham raise beginning position

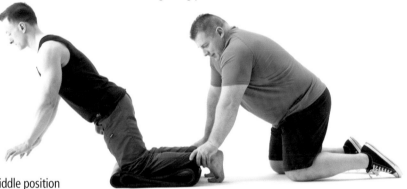

Glute ham raise middle position

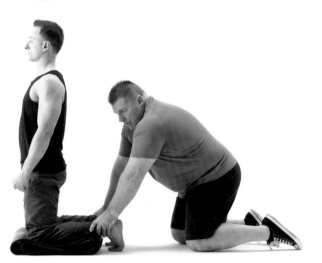

Glute ham raise finish position

# The Single Leg Calf Raise

To begin, step one foot onto a small platform that is 4 to 6 inches high. Only the front half of your foot should remain on the platform. Now, squeeze your calf muscle and raise your heel straight up into the air. You should feel a strong contraction in the calf. Now lower your heel until you feel a slight stretch. Repeat the movement. Complete all of the required repetitions on one leg before switching to the other leg.

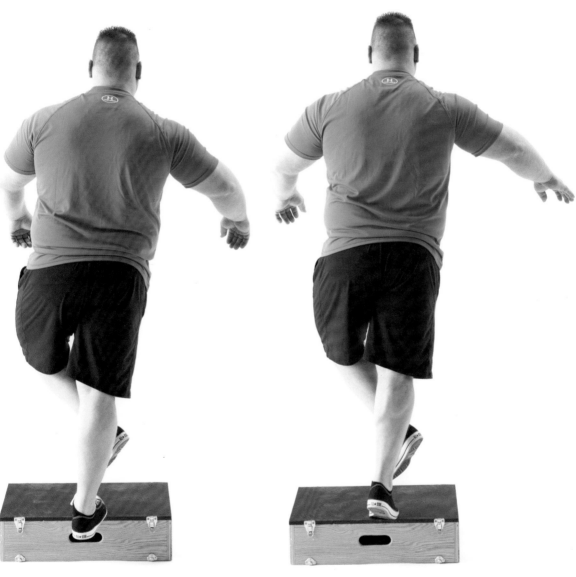

Single leg calf raise beginning position          Single leg calf raise finish position

# Bodyweight Grinds Upper Body

## Neuro-Grip Push-Up

To perform this exercise you will need a pair of Neuro-Grips. This style of push-up has been around for quite a while. They are sometimes referred to as iron cross, T-grip , or spike handle push-ups. The Neuro-Grip is a variation of the many T-shaped push-up handles. Using the Neuro-Grips increases the intensity of the push-up exercise. Neuro-Grip push-ups work the whole body to work as a unit, increasing neuromuscular efficiency. Begin by grasping the Neuro-Grips and placing your body into the top position of a push-up. Keeping your elbows close to your sides slowly lower your body until your chest is around 4 to 6 inches away from the floor. Pause for a moment, then slowly raise up to the top position. Repeat the exercise for the required amount of repetitions.

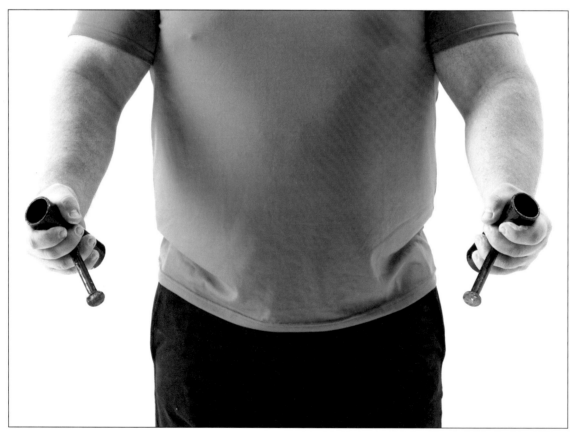

Neuro-Grips

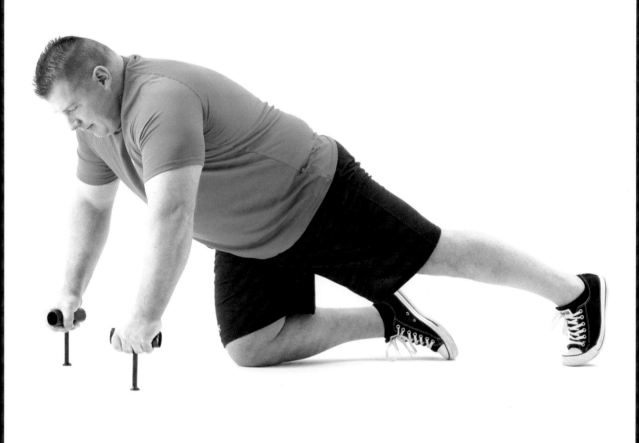

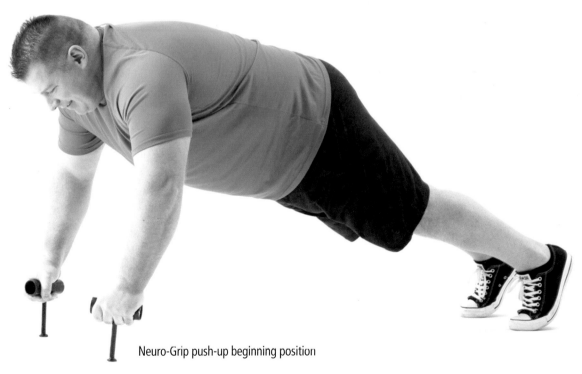

Neuro-Grip push-up beginning position

**Performance Point:** Focus on tensing the abdominals and crushing the Neuro-Grips throughout the entire movement.

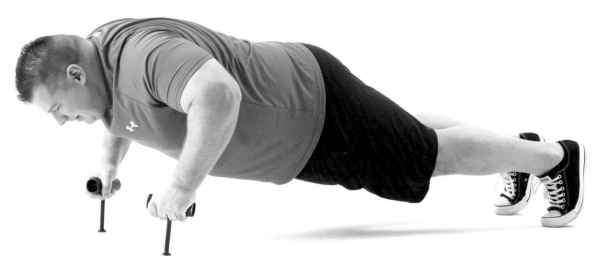

Neuro-Grip push-up middle position

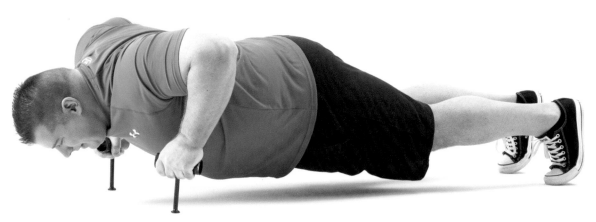

Neuro-Grip push-up finish position

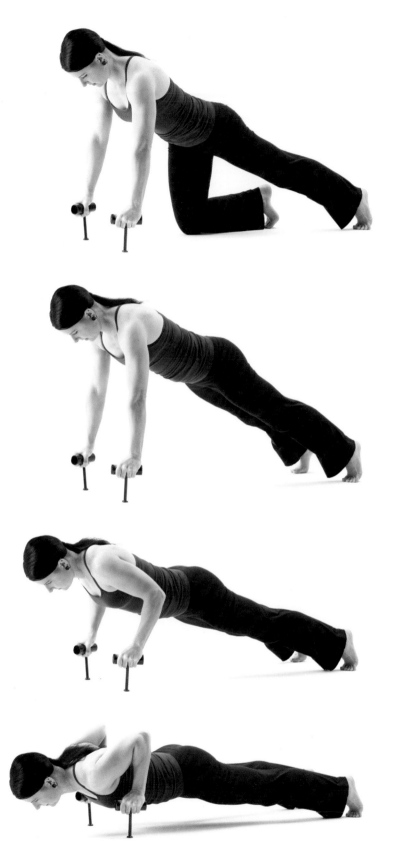

# Handstand Push-Ups

The handstand push-up is one of the best mass and strength building exercises in the Neuro-Mass arsenal. This exercise has been a staple in the workout programs of the old-time strongman, martial artist, acrobats, and many others. Because handstand push-ups require inversion, the lymphatic system is stimulated and there is increased blood flow to the brain.

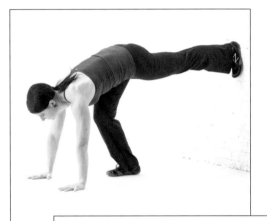

The technique we will use to get into position for the handstand push-up, is called "wall walking." To begin, place both feet flat against a wall, while your hands and knees are on the floor. Now, driving your hands into the floor, begin to walk up the wall using your hands and feet. Make sure to contract the abdominals throughout the movement. When you reach the top position, slowly lower your body until your head is a few inches away from the floor. Pause for a moment and raise your body up to the top position. Repeat the exercise for the required amount of repetitions before wall walking down to the floor.

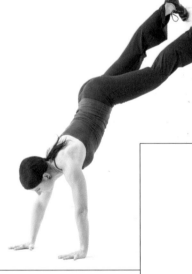

Wall walk progression

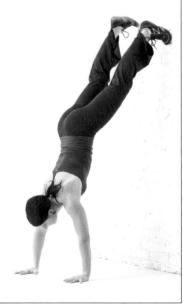

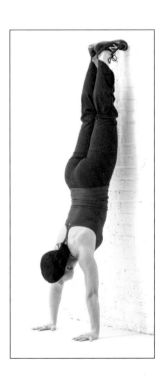

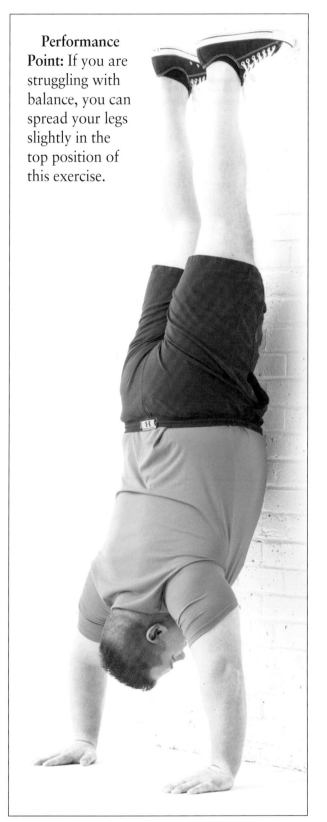

**Performance Point:** If you are struggling with balance, you can spread your legs slightly in the top position of this exercise.

Handstand push-up lockout position

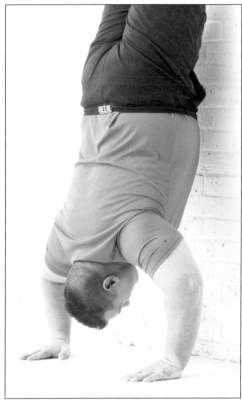

Handstand push-up middle position

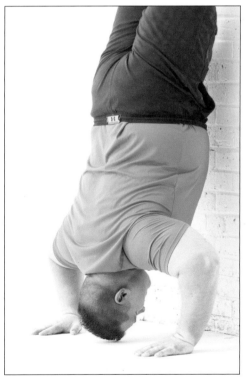

Handstand push-up lower position

129

## Shoulder Levers

This movement creates incredibly powerful shoulders. To begin this exercise, lie on your side with your upper arm tucked under you. Your elbows should be bent and your forearm should be perpendicular to your body. Now, pressurize the core and lift your body off the floor by driving the elbow and forearm into the floor. The range of motion of this exercise is very short.

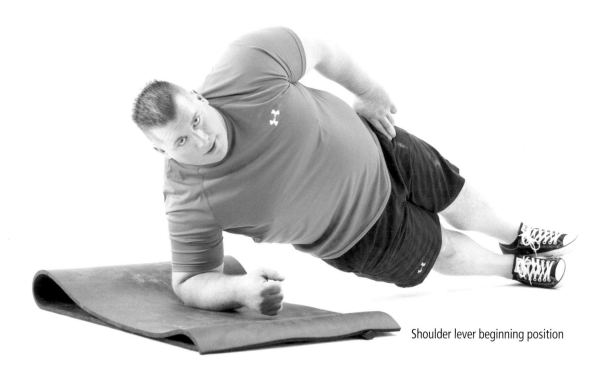

Shoulder lever beginning position

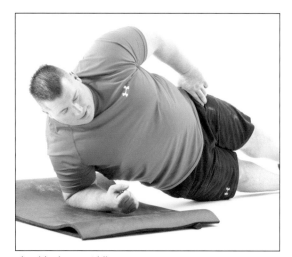

Shoulder lever middle position

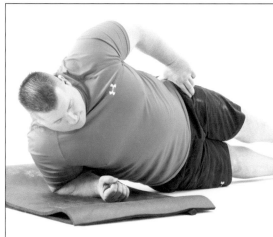

Shoulder lever finish position

# Incline Wall Push-Ups

Incline wall push-ups elevate the feet creating leverage, which makes the push-up more difficult. Begin by performing the wall walk. Stop when your feet are halfway up the wall. Keeping your back straight and your abdominals tensed, slowly lower your body toward the floor. Stop when your chest is 4 to 6 inches away from the floor. Pause for a moment and slowly push your body away from the ground until you're in the starting position. Repeat the exercise for the required amount of repetitions before wall walking down to the floor.

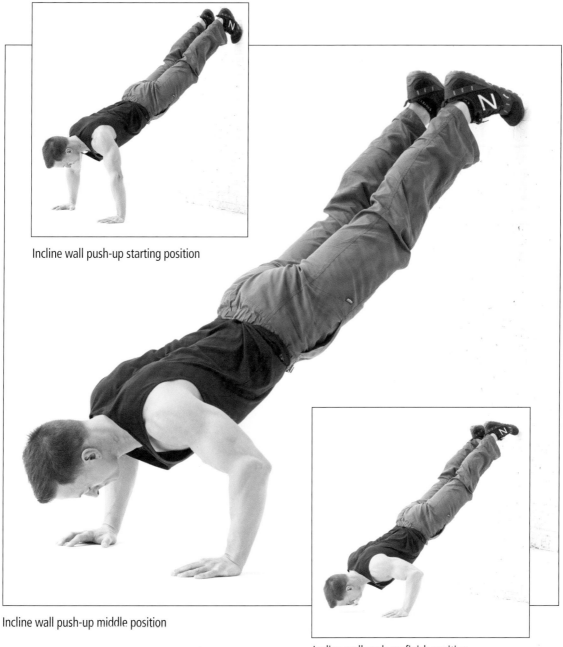

Incline wall push-up starting position

Incline wall push-up middle position

Incline wall push-up finish position

# Sledgehammer Push-Ups

To perform this exercise you will need two sledgehammers. Place the hammers with the heads on the floor and the handles pointing straight up. Grasp the hammer handles about halfway up.

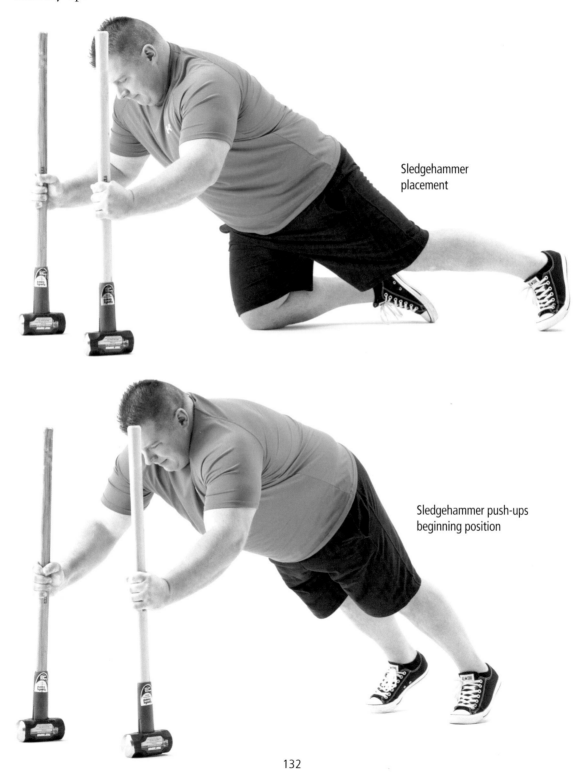

Sledgehammer placement

Sledgehammer push-ups beginning position

Now, step both legs back until you are in the top position of the push-up. Crushing the handles and squeezing the abdominals, slowly lower your upper body until you feel your biceps meet your forearms. Pause for a moment and slowly raise to the starting position. Repeat the exercise for the required amount of repetitions. Sledgehammer push-ups will develop powerful wrists and a bone crushing grip.

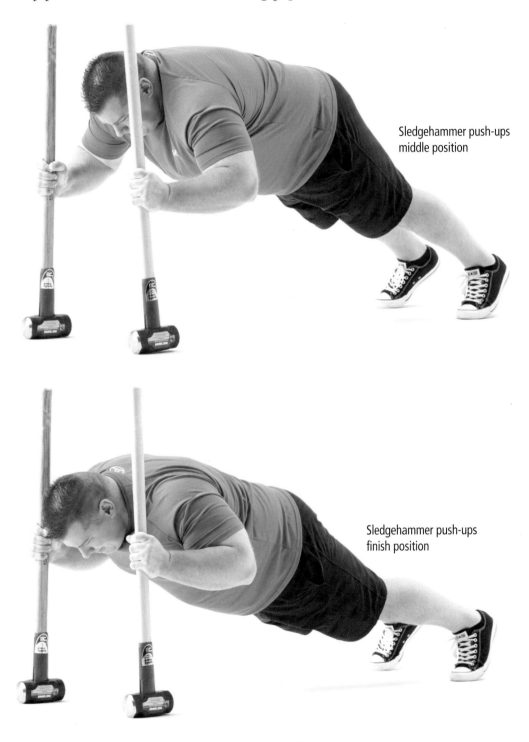

Sledgehammer push-ups
middle position

Sledgehammer push-ups
finish position

# Chest Elevated Push-Ups

This exercise requires a small step or platform around 12 inches high. Place both hands on the platform. Now, step both feet back into the push-up position. Squeezing the core, slowly lower your body until your chest is around 4 to 6 inches away from the platform. Pause for a moment and slowly return to the starting position. Repeat this movement for the required amount of repetitions.

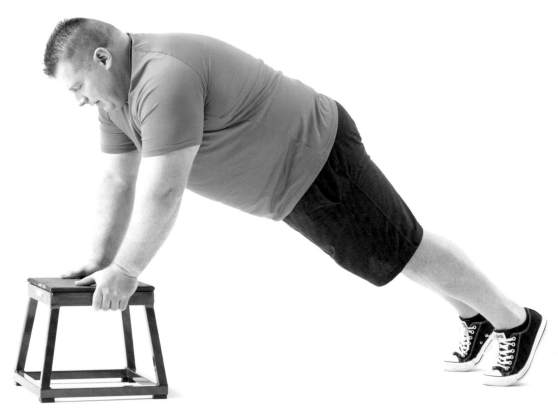

Chest elevated push-up progression with side grip

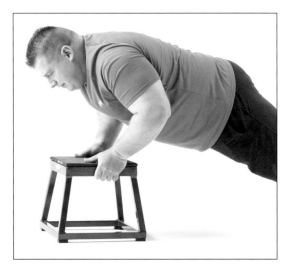
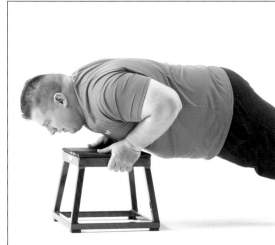

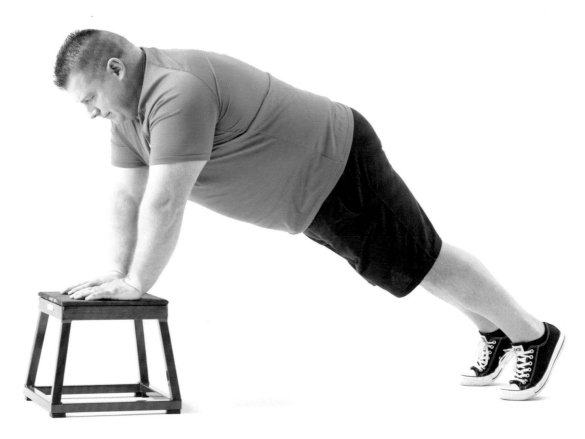

Chest elevated push-up progression with flat palms

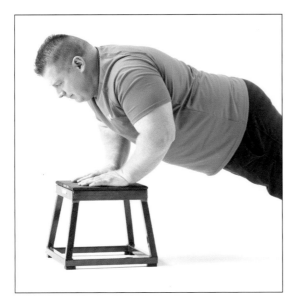
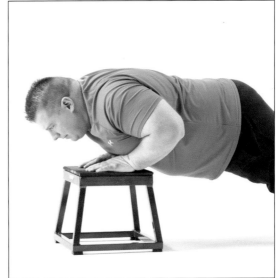

# Medicine Ball Crush Push-Ups

To perform this exercise you will need a medicine ball. To begin, place a medicine ball on the floor. Now, grasp the sides of the medicine ball with your hands at chest level. Crushing the ball with your hands, step both feet back until you are in the top of the push-up position. Using whole body tension, slowly lower yourself until your chest is almost touching the ball. Pause for a moment and slowly return to the starting position. Repeat the exercise for the required amount of repetitions.

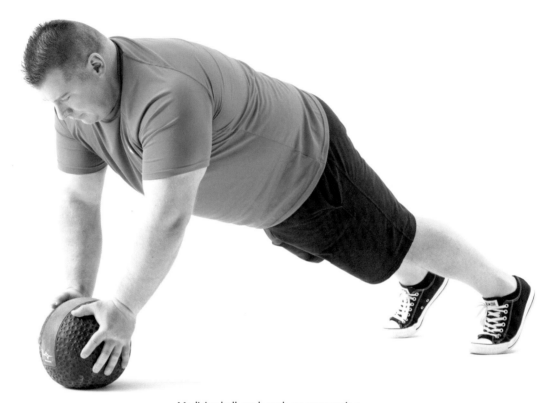

Medicine ball crush push-up progression

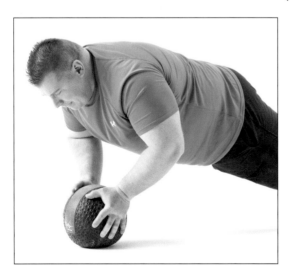
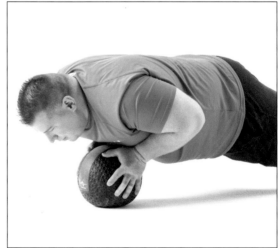

# One Arm Supported Push-Ups

This exercise requires the use of a small step 8 to 10 inches high or a medicine ball. Place one hand on medicine ball and the opposite hand on the floor as you get into the top position of a push-up. Tensing the body, slowly lower yourself until your chest is around 6 inches above the floor. Pause for a moment, and slowly raise your body to the starting position. Repeat all the required amount of repetitions on one side before moving to the opposite side.

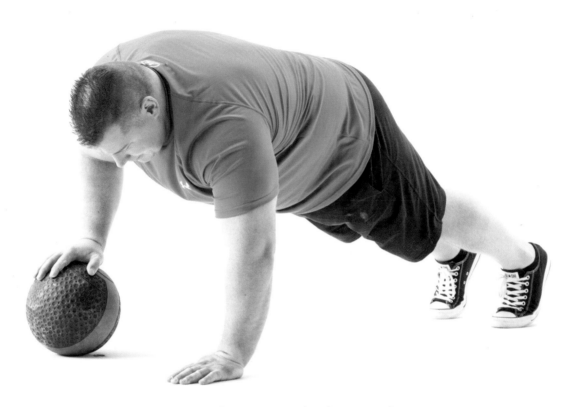

One arm supported push-up progression

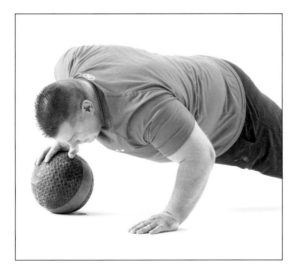
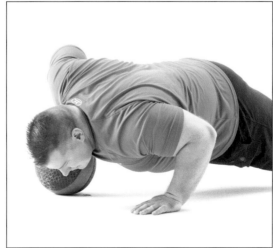

137

## The Inverted Bodyweight Row

This exercise requires the use of a low pull up bar. You may substitute gymnastic rings, a heavy-duty desk, or even a bar resting on the top of two chairs. The bar should be at least waist high. Lay on your back underneath the bar, so that it is over your chest. Reach up and grasp the bar with an overhand grip. Now, tense the abdominals and squeeze the bar as you pull yourself up. Drive your elbows back and squeeze the shoulder blades together until your chest touches the bar. Pause for a moment, and slowly lower yourself to the starting position. Repeat this exercise for the required amount of repetitions.

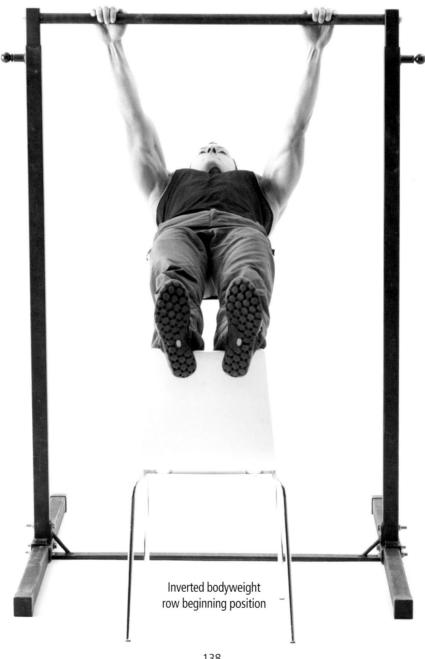

Inverted bodyweight
row beginning position

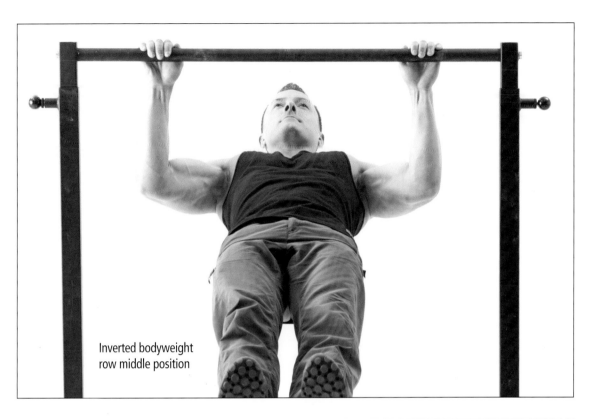

Inverted bodyweight
row middle position

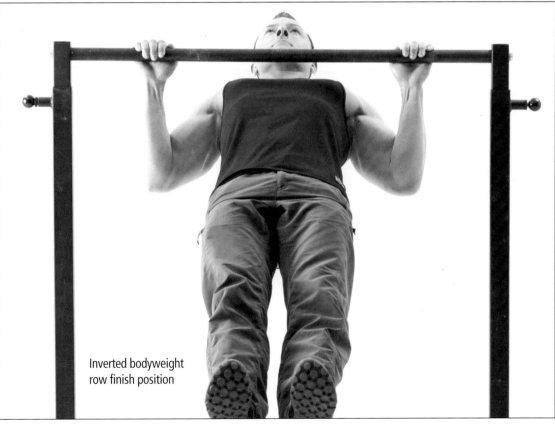

Inverted bodyweight
row finish position

# The Single Leg Shoulder Bridge

Begin by lying on your back. Both arms should lay at your sides. Bend one knee and straighten out the opposite leg. Now, drive with your foot and raise your hips into the air. Pause for a moment and lower to the starting position. Repeat the required amount of repetitions on one leg before moving to the opposite leg.

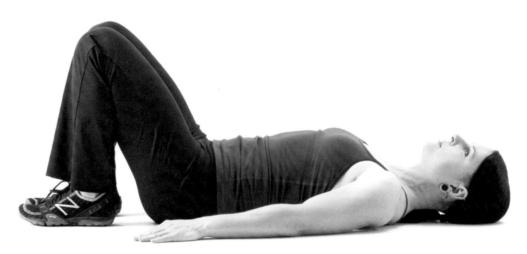

Single leg shoulder bridge beginning position

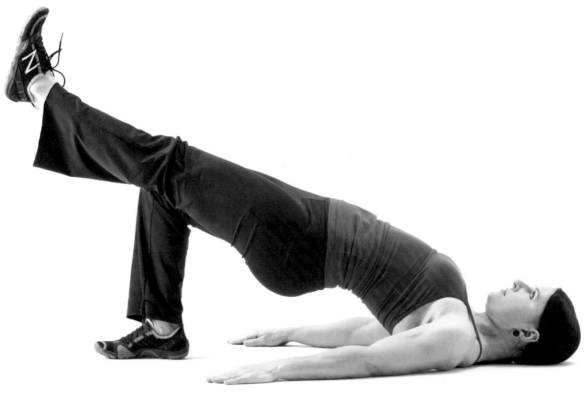

Single leg shoulder bridge finish position

# Pull Ups

This exercise requires the use of a pull up bar. Grasp the bar with an overhand grip. Your hands should be slightly beyond shoulder width. Crushing the bar and squeezing the abdominals, slowly pull yourself up until your chin is above the bar. Pause for a moment, and slowly lower yourself down to the starting position. Repeat the exercise for the required amount of repetitions.

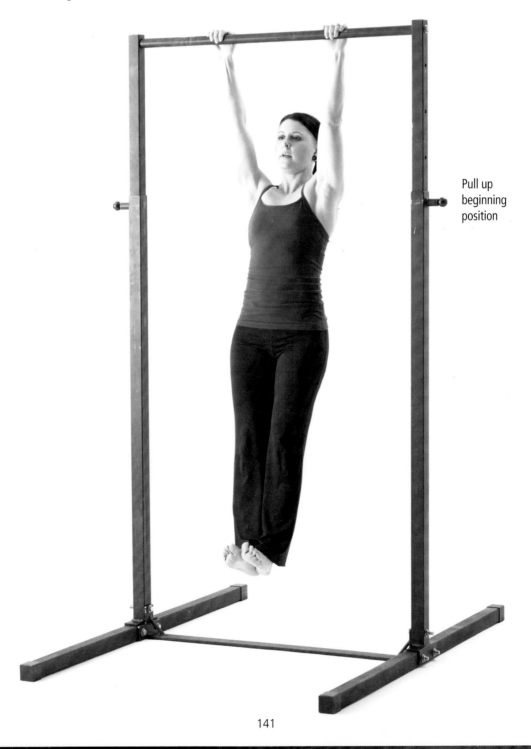

Pull up beginning position

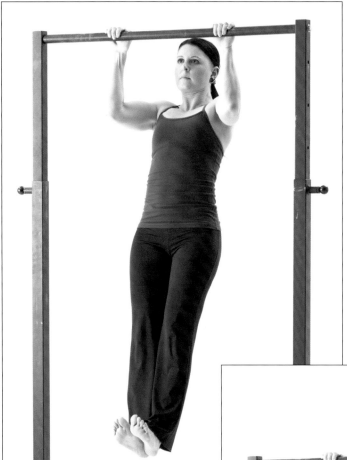

Pull up middle position

Pull up finish position

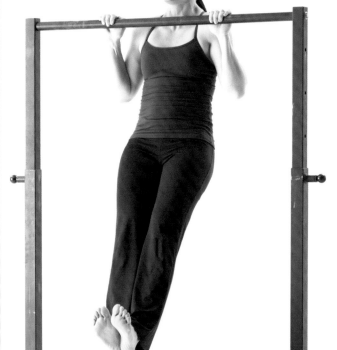

142

## The Hanging Leg Raise

To perform this exercise you will need a pull up bar. Grasp the bar with an overhand grip and hands shoulder width apart. Hinging at the hips, raise your legs until they are perpendicular with your body. Try to keep your legs straight as possible. Pause for a moment and slowly lower your legs to the starting position. Repeat the exercise for the required amount of repetitions.

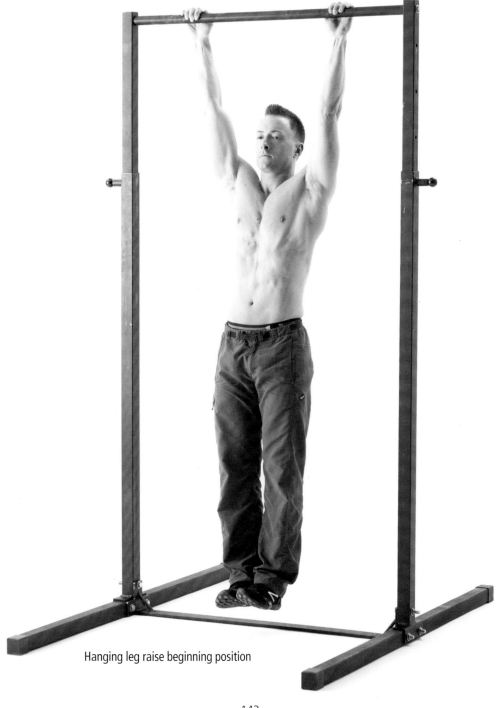

Hanging leg raise beginning position

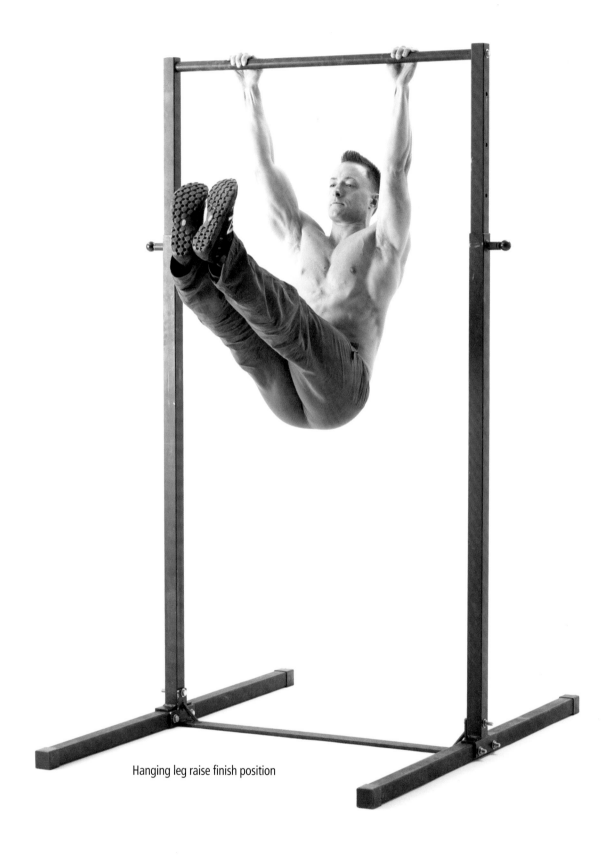

Hanging leg raise finish position

## The Inverted Bodyweight Row Position Claw Curl

This exercise begins just like the inverted bodyweight row, except you only grasp the bar with your fingertips. Keeping your arms straight, pull your body upwards using your fingertips to pull the bar into the palm. Pause for a moment and slowly lower to the starting position.

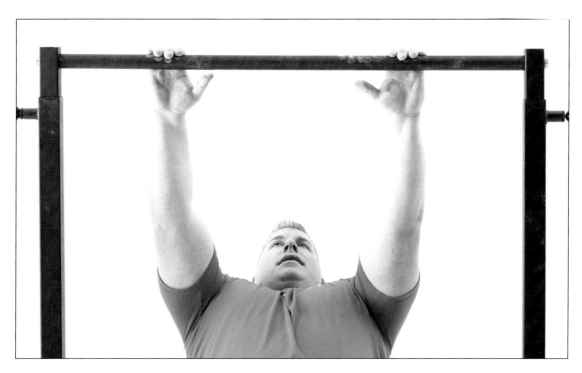

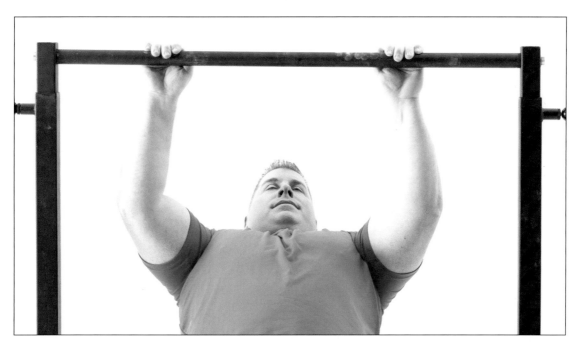

# Dynamic Power Drills Lower Body

## Anchor Sprints

Bring your arms to chest level and lock them straight out. Holding a standard yoga block between your palms, press both of your thumbs together until you feel your chest muscles are activated. Now, began an all-out sprint. This biomechanical advantage exercise will increase your speed, power, and neuromuscular efficiency. Continue sprinting for the required amount of time.

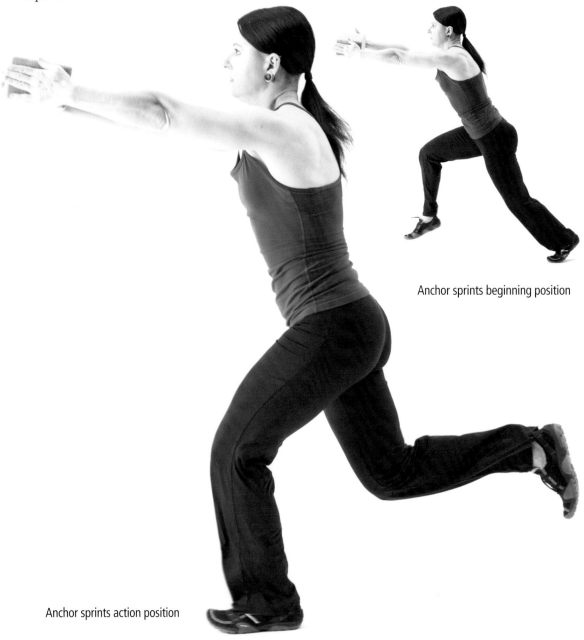

Anchor sprints beginning position

Anchor sprints action position

# Arms Overhead Sprints

Lock out both arms straight up into the air. Your fingers should be pointed upward. Now begin an all-out sprint. Continue running for the required amount of time.

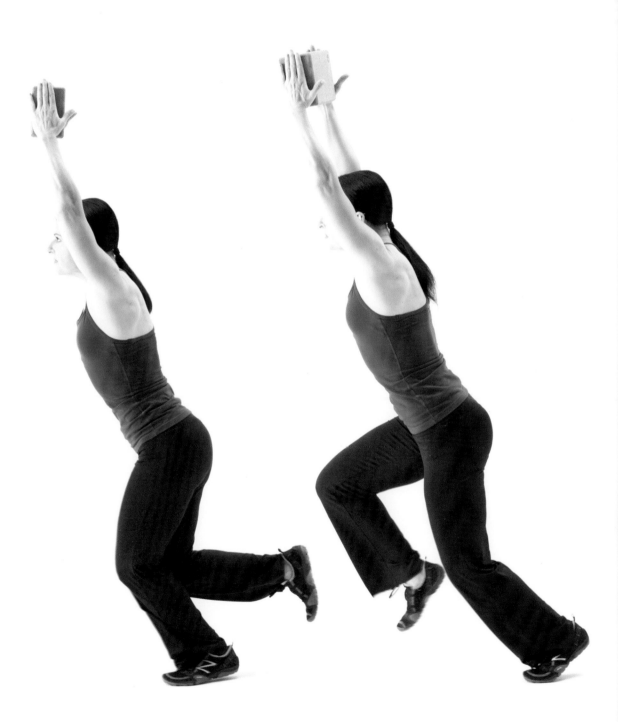

## Mule Kicks

To begin, lower your upper body into a squat. From this position, fall forward onto your hands. Driving your hands into the ground, explosively kick your feet high into the air. You should land on the balls of your feet. Continue this kicking motion for the required amount of time.

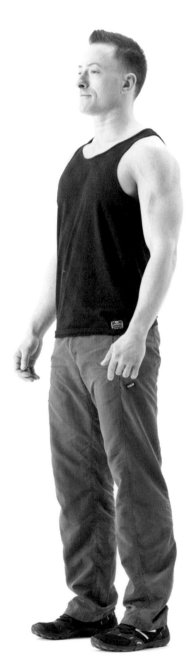

Mule kick beginning/finish position

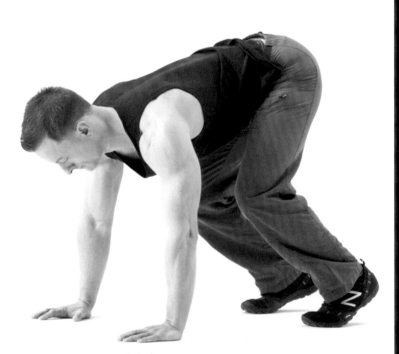

Mule kick squat position

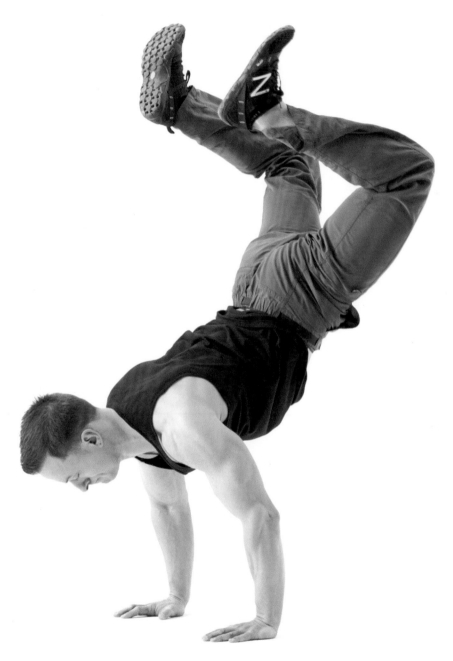

Mule kick airborne position

# Explosive Lunges

To begin, lock out both arms straight up into the air. Keeping your back straight, step one leg behind you until you are into a lunge position. Now, explosively drive your body straight into the air. While airborne, switch legs so that the rear leg is now in the front lunge position. Repeat this exercise for the required amount of time.

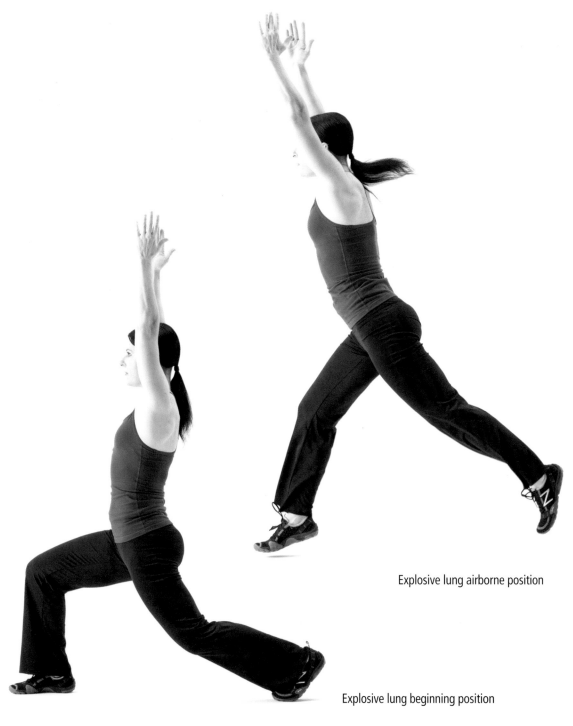

Explosive lung airborne position

Explosive lung beginning position

# Jump Squats

Start by placing your feet shoulder width apart. Now, lower yourself into a squat. When you reach the bottom position, drive your feet through the floor and explode straight up until you are airborne. Land on the balls of your feet, and repeat the exercise for the required amount of time.

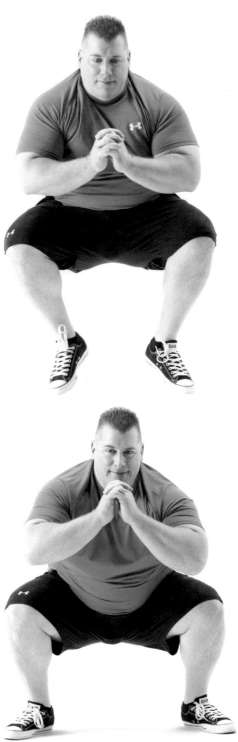

Jump squats airborne position

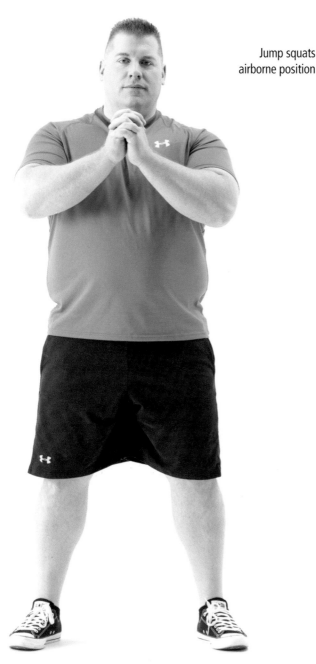

Jump squats beginning position

Jump squats finish position

# The Lateral Shuffle

To begin, squat down until your thighs are slightly above parallel position to the ground. Pushing off your left foot, began to shuffle your body to the right. After three or more repetitions, push off with your right foot and shuffle your body to the left. Change directions every 3 to 5 repetitions. Repeat the exercise for the required amount of time.

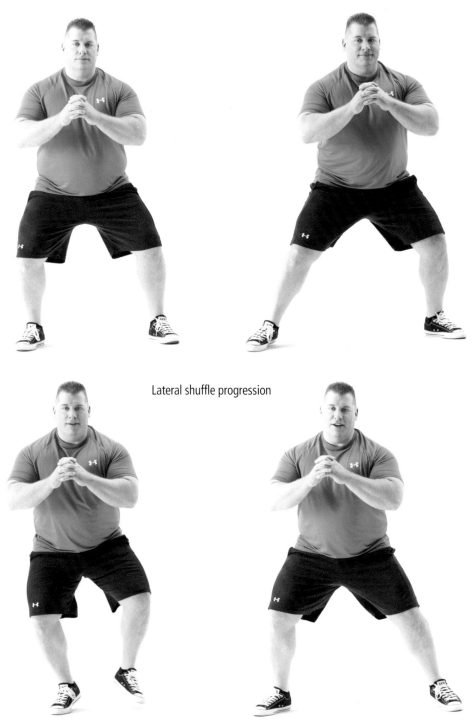

Lateral shuffle progression

## The Broad Jump

The exercise begins by dropping your body into a partial squat. Now, explosively drive your feet into the ground and propel yourself forward. Try to cover as much distance as you can with every jump. Continue this movement for the required amount of time.

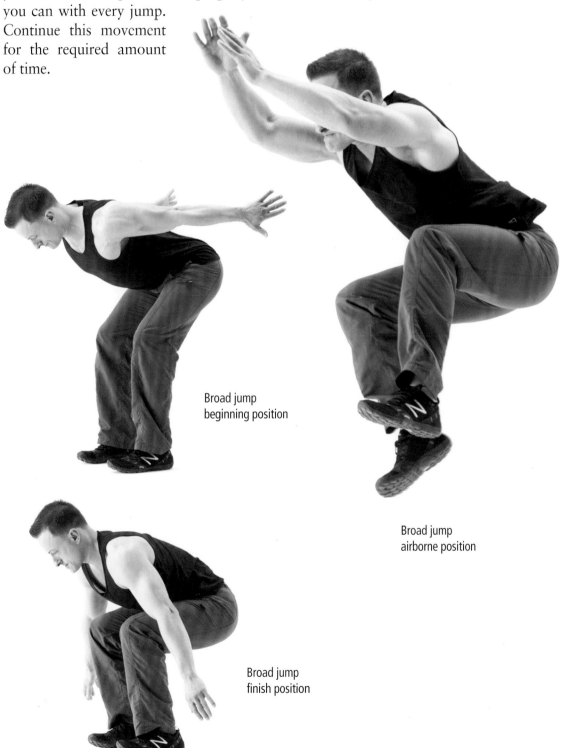

Broad jump beginning position

Broad jump airborne position

Broad jump finish position

# Hanging Lower Body Catch and Throw

This exercise requires the use of a pull up bar, medicine ball, and a partner. Grasp a pull up bar with an overhand grip and allow your legs to hang freely. Now, have a partner toss the medicine ball to you as you try to catch it with your feet.

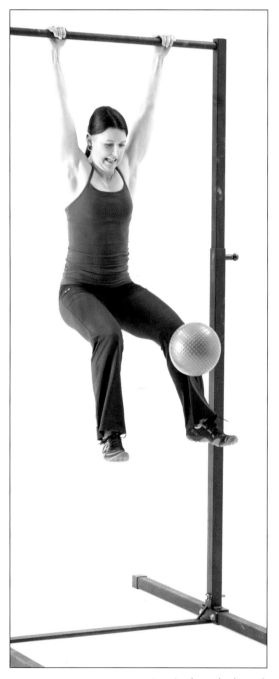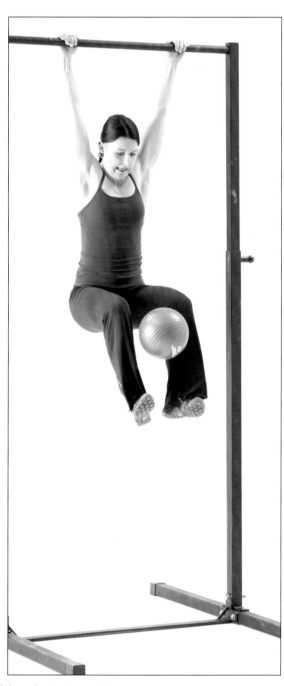

Hanging lower body catch and throw beginning position

After you have caught the ball, throw the ball back to your partner using your feet. Continue this catching and throwing exercise for the required amount of time.

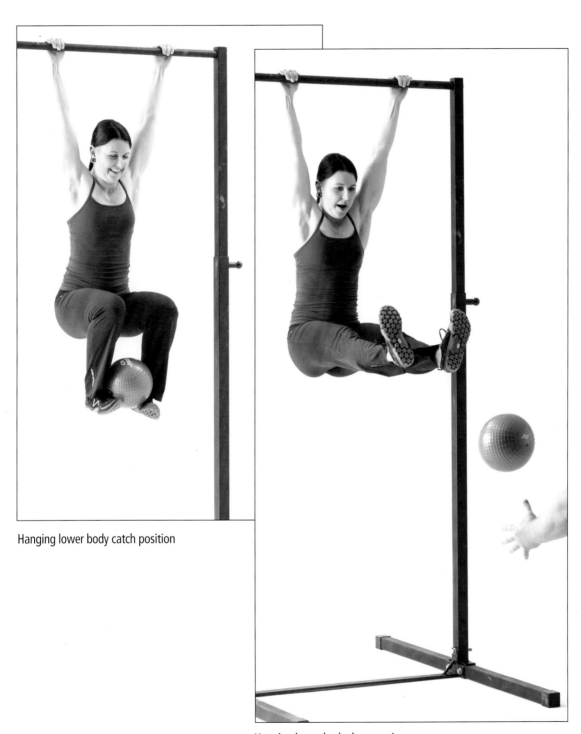

Hanging lower body catch position

Hanging lower body throw action

# The Platform Jump

To perform this exercise you will need a step or platform that is 12 inches tall or higher and can support your body weight. Stand from the platform with your feet shoulder width apart. Squat down and explosively jump into the air until the balls of your feet land on the platform. Now, jump backwards off the platform landing on the balls of your feet. This exercise should be performed as rapidly and explosively as possible. Continue jumping for the required amount of time.

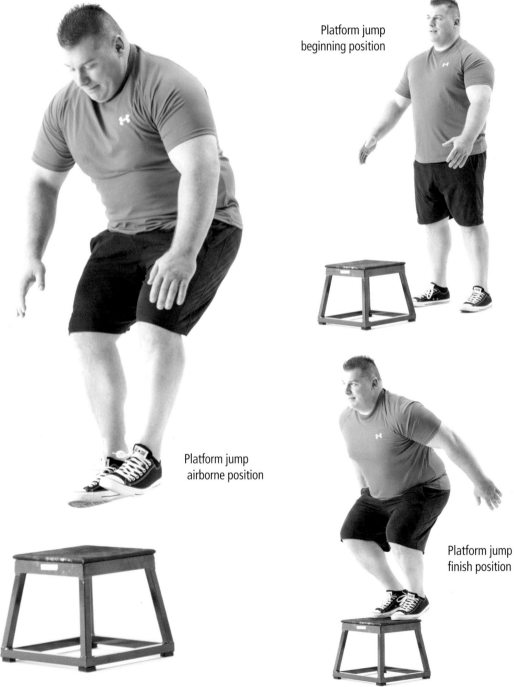

Platform jump
beginning position

Platform jump
airborne position

Platform jump
finish position

## Lateral Hops

This exercise requires the use of an implement to hop over. An agility cone, kettlebell, or medicine ball would be good choices for this movement. Stand to the left of your implement, squat down slightly and explosively hop laterally by pushing off with your left foot. As you begin to be airborne, pull your knees up so that your feet clear the implement below. Land on the balls of your feet. Now repeat the movement, by explosively hopping and pushing off with the right foot. This exercise should be performed as rapidly and explosively as possible. Continue hopping for the required amount of time.

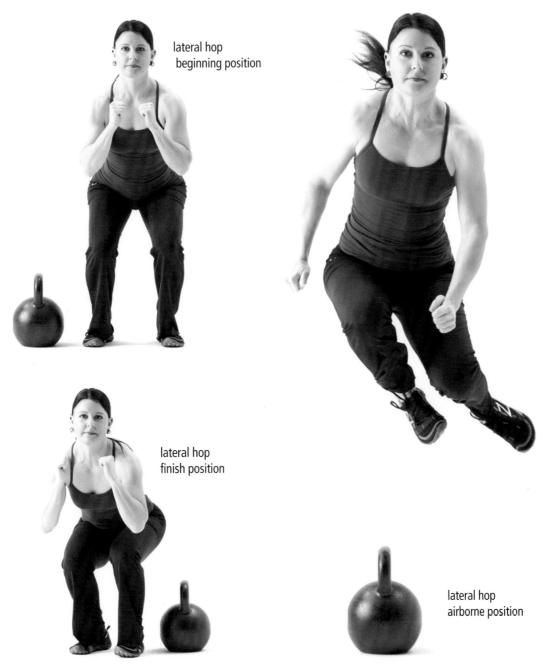

lateral hop
beginning position

lateral hop
finish position

lateral hop
airborne position

# Bodyweight Reverse Hyperextensions

To begin, find a table or bench that is higher than your hips. Place your upper body from your waist up face down on the bench. Your hips should hinge on the end of the bench. Explosively drive your heels backwards until your body is completely straight. Now, let the legs swing down to the starting position. Repeat this movement for the required amount of time.

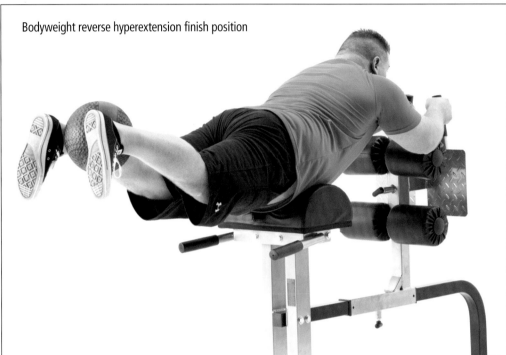

Bodyweight reverse hyperextension finish position

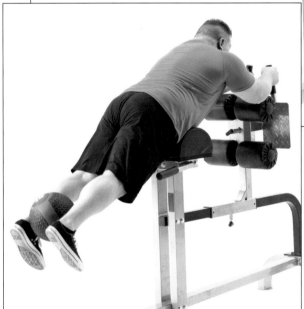

Bodyweight reverse hyperextension middle position

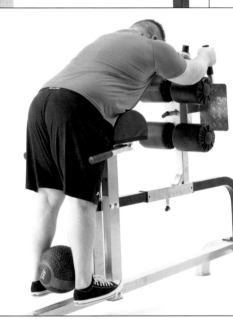

Bodyweight reverse hyperextension beginning position

## Wall Hops

   Start by facing a wall and raise your hands over your head. Now, with a slight bend in your knees, use your calves to explosively jump straight up. As you become airborne reach and touch the wall at the highest point in your jump with your hands. Repeat this movement for the required amount of time.

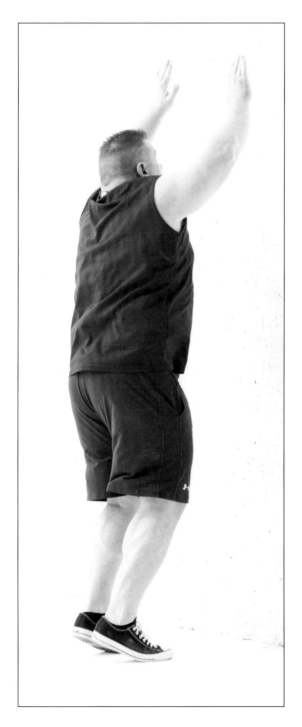
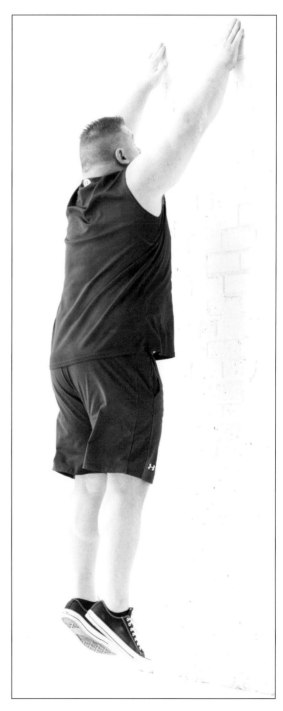

## Bootstrappers

To begin this exercise, get into a six-point stance on the floor—meaning your toes, knees, and hands are all touching the ground. Pushing off with your hands, raise your hips up into the air until your legs have straightened out. Walk your hands slightly back, and allow the knees to bend down into a squatting position before repeating the exercise. Continue this movement for the required amount of time.

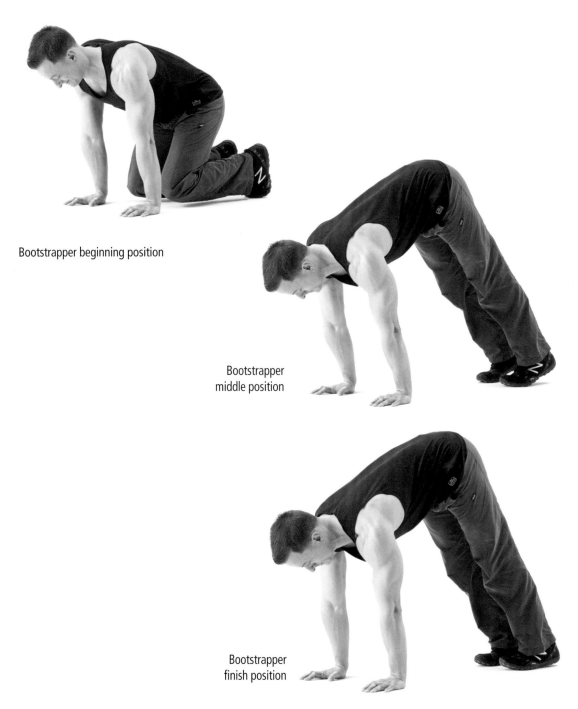

Bootstrapper beginning position

Bootstrapper middle position

Bootstrapper finish position

# Dynamic Power Drills Upper Body

## Double Strike Push-Ups

Begin by placing your body into the top position of the push-up. Lower your body into the bottom position of the push-up.

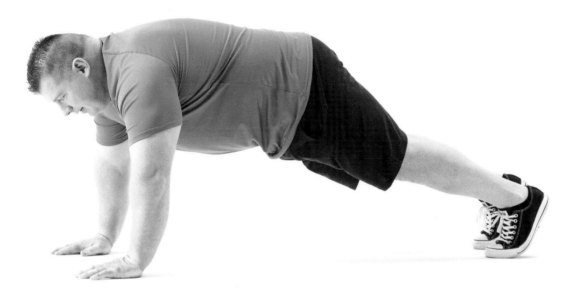

Double strike push-up beginning position

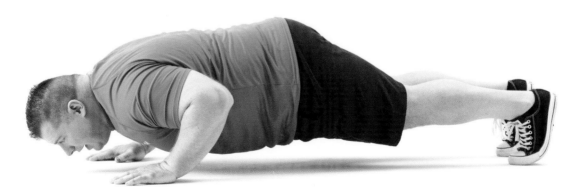

Double strike push-up lower position

Explosively push off the floor until your upper body is airborne. Now, strike the ground with the right palm followed by the left. Finish all repetitions on the right hand lead before leading with the left hand. If you are doing this exercise correctly you will hear a rhythmic slap-slap sound. Repeat the exercise for the required amount of time.

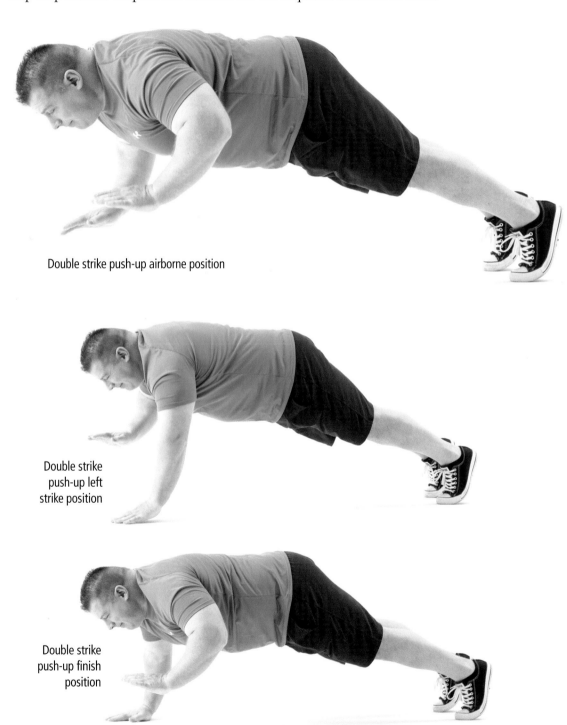

Double strike push-up airborne position

Double strike push-up left strike position

Double strike push-up finish position

# Floor Fire Push-Ups

This exercise has a very short range of motion and should be performed explosively. Begin by placing your body in the top position of the push-up. With a slight flex in your elbows explosively power your body upward. Upon landing, only allow a slight flex in the elbow before repeating the movement. The goal of the exercise is for your hands to touch the floor for as little time as possible. Imagine that floor is on fire. Remember to keep the range of motion short. Repeat this exercise for the required amount of time.

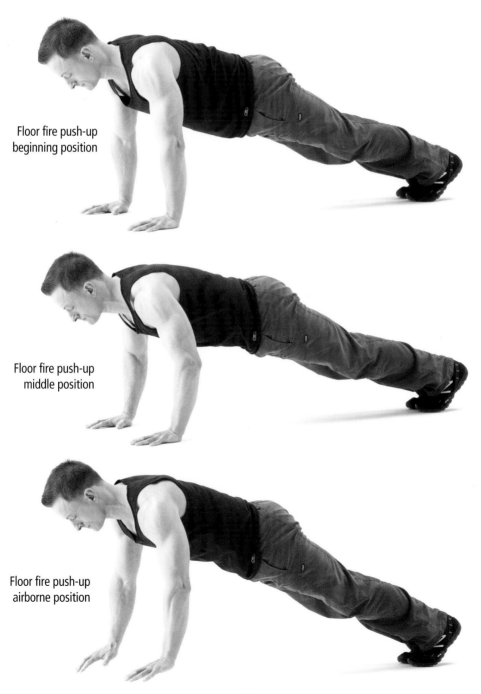

Floor fire push-up
beginning position

Floor fire push-up
middle position

Floor fire push-up
airborne position

# Medicine Ball/Basketball Bouncing Push-Ups

To perform this exercise you will need a rubber medicine ball or heavy duty basketball. To begin, place the medicine ball on the floor. Now, grasp the sides of the medicine ball with your hands at chest level. Crushing the ball with your hands, step both feet back until you are in the top of the push-up position. Now, with a slight bend in the elbows explosively press upwards until the ball becomes airborne. Upon landing, immediately repeat the movement. Continue this bouncing movement for the required amount of time.

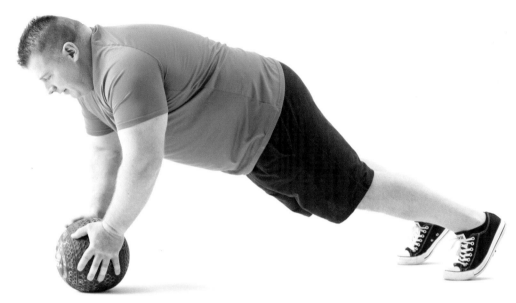

Medicine ball bouncing push-ups beginning position

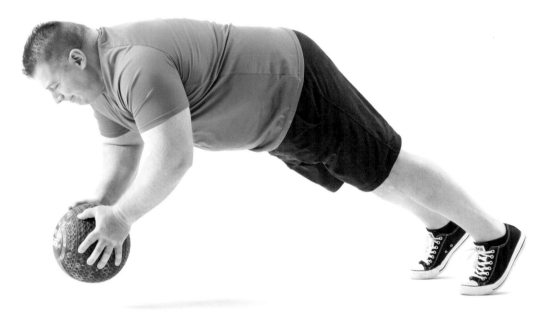

Medicine ball bouncing push-ups airborne position

# The Hummingbird

Begin by placing your arms straight out at your sides and lower into a semi-squat position. Now, explosively move your arms up and down within a 6-inch range of motion. The range of motion is extremely small. You'll find that this innovative exercise has the ability to fatigue shoulders very quickly. To increase balance and athleticism, this exercise can be performed on one leg. Repeat the movement for the required amount of time.

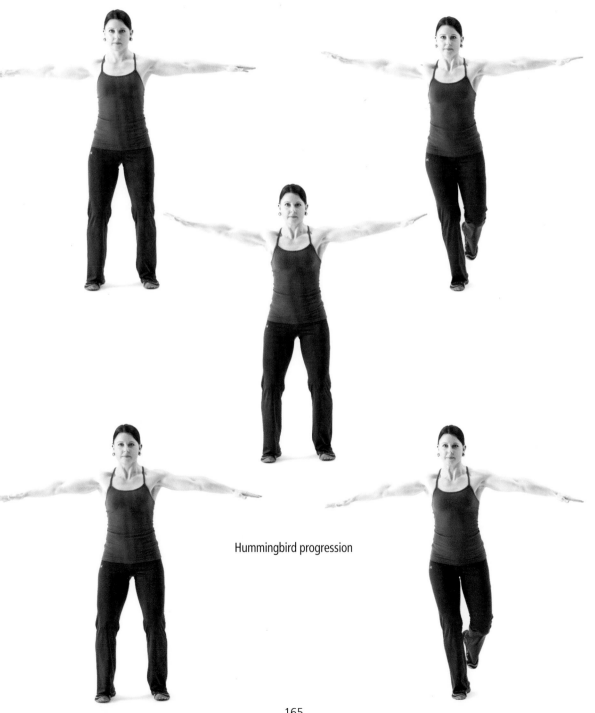

Hummingbird progression

# Seated Arm Sprints

Start by sitting on the floor with your legs together straight out in front of you. Now, bend your elbows so they form a 90° angle. With your elbows locked in place, raise your right arm until your fist is at chin level while simultaneously driving your left arm backward. Now, explosively reverse the movement. Continue this rapid pumping action for the required amount of time.

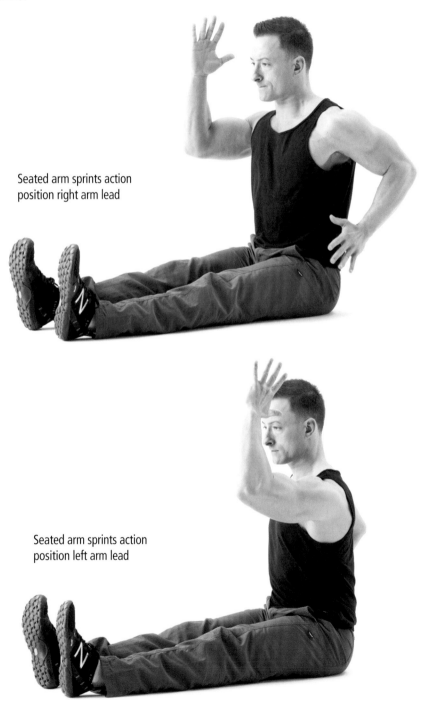

Seated arm sprints action position right arm lead

Seated arm sprints action position left arm lead

# The Inverted Speed Row

For this exercise you will need a low hanging pull up bar and a sturdy towel or nylon strap. Lay on your back so that the bar is perpendicular to your body. Reach up and grasp the towel ends with your hands. Now, pull down with your right hand as you allow the left hand to rise up. Immediately reverse the movement. The exercise should feel like you are performing reverse punches. Perform this exercise as rapidly and explosively as possible. Repeat this movement for the required amount of time.

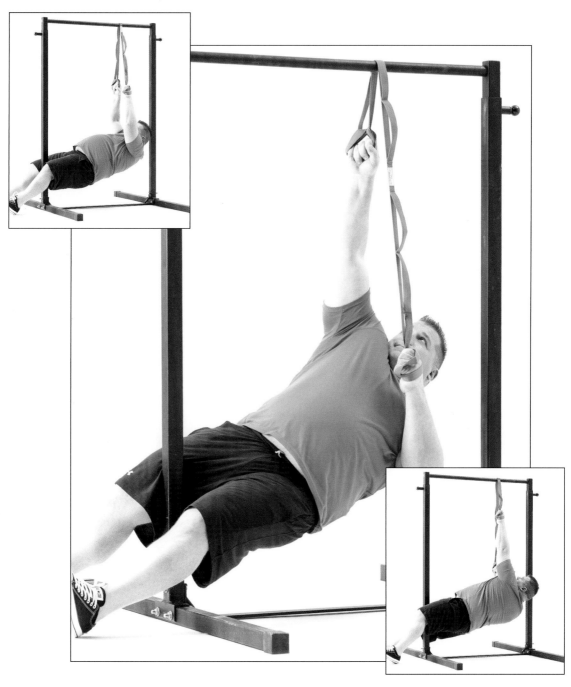

# Heavy Bag Speed Punches

To perform this exercise, you will need a heavy bag. You may also use a wall if you wear padded boxing gloves. With your feet shoulder length apart rapidly punch the bag at chest level. Alternate hands with every punch. Try to make these punches as explosive as possible. Repeat this movement for the required amount of time.

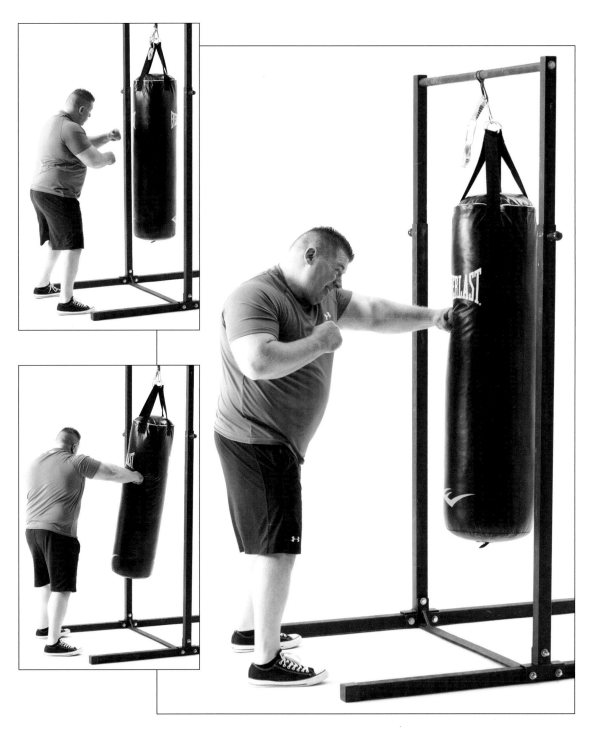

## Lateral Moving Step Push-Ups

This exercise requires the use of a step or box at least 12 inches high. Begin by placing your right hand on the step and your left hand on the floor as you position your body to perform a push-up. Now, drop down into the lower portion of the push-up. Explosively push your body into the air laterally so that your left hand will land on the step and your right hand on the floor. Reverse the movement and repeat the exercise for the required amount of time. To make this exercise easier, simply walk with your hands laterally over the step and perform a push-up.

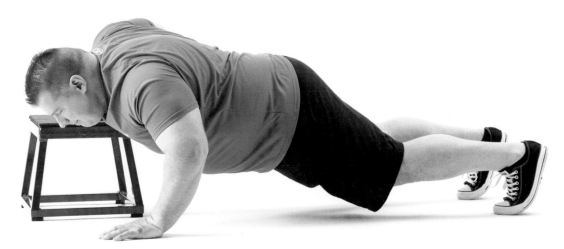

Lateral moving step push-up beginning position

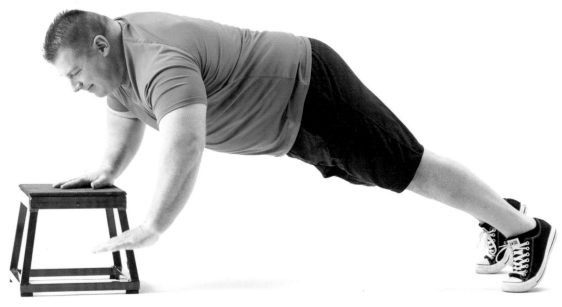

Lateral moving step push-up left hand down position

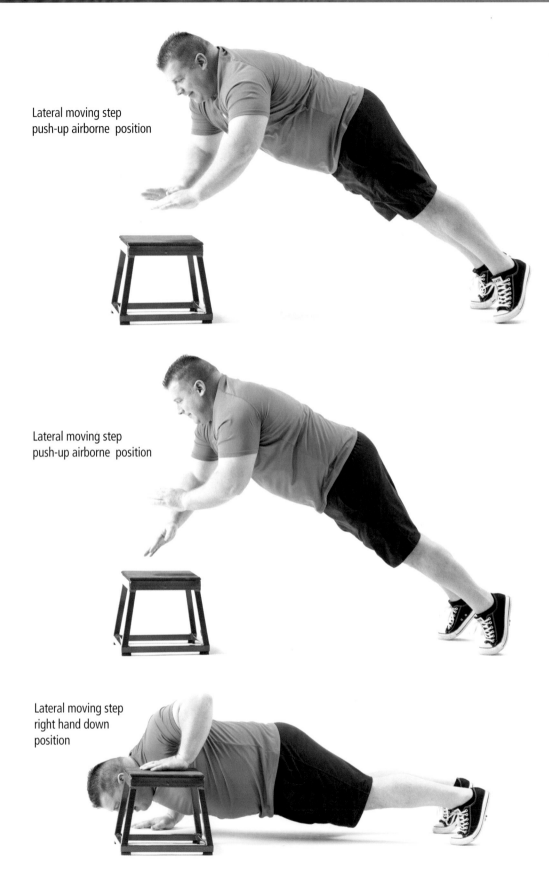

Lateral moving step
push-up airborne position

Lateral moving step
push-up airborne position

Lateral moving step
right hand down
position

170

# The Treadmill Hand Crawl

To perform this exercise you will need a treadmill. Begin by raising the incline of a treadmill to its highest level. Now, adjust the speed according to your ability. Place both feet on the floor and your hands on the treadmill belt as you begin crawling using only your hands. Continue this movement for the required amount of time.

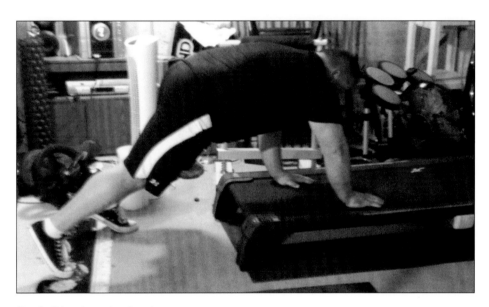

Treadmill hand crawl action shot

# The Pull Up Bar Walk

This exercise requires the use of a pull up bar. Stand on the far end of a pull up bar so that it is perpendicular to your body. Now, grasp the bar with both hands in an overhand grip with one hand in front of the other. Both thumbs should be pointing toward you. Begin to walk the length of the bar by placing one hand in front of the other until you reach the end. Now, reverse the movement by walking the hands backwards. Repeat the movement for the required amount of time.

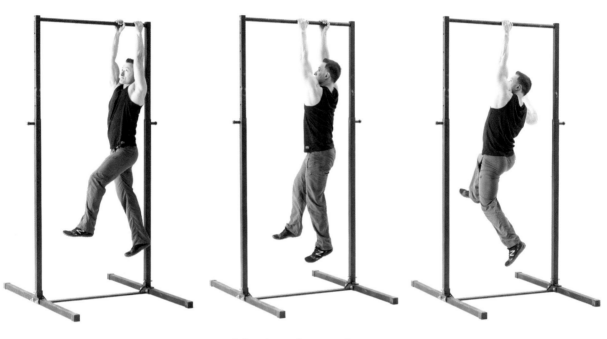

Pull up bar walk progression

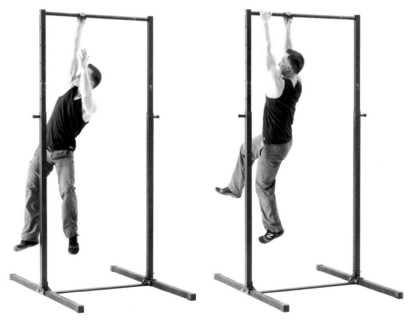

172

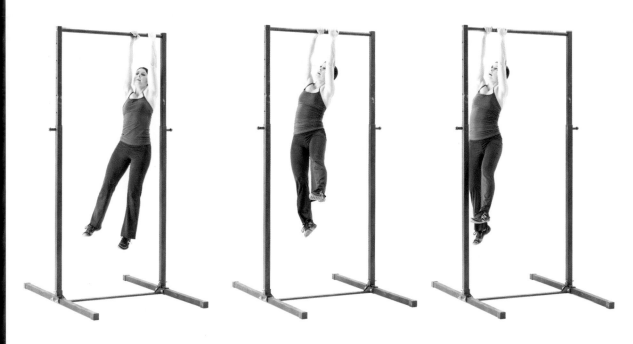

Pull up bar walk progression

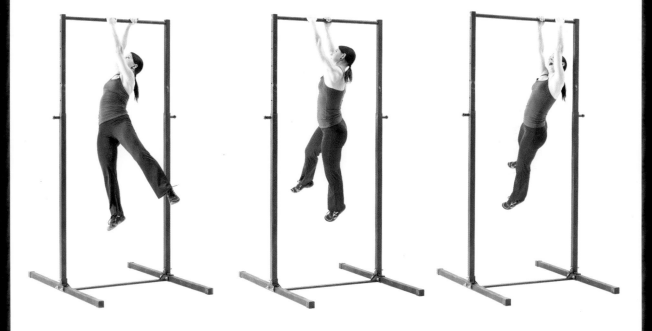

# Russian Twists

To begin, sit on the floor with knees bent and both hands clasped together with elbows tight to the sides. Slightly lean back so that your feet are off the floor and your weight is supported on your glutes. Now, rotate your hands to the right as you rotate your knees to the left. Reverse the movement and repeat for the required amount of time.

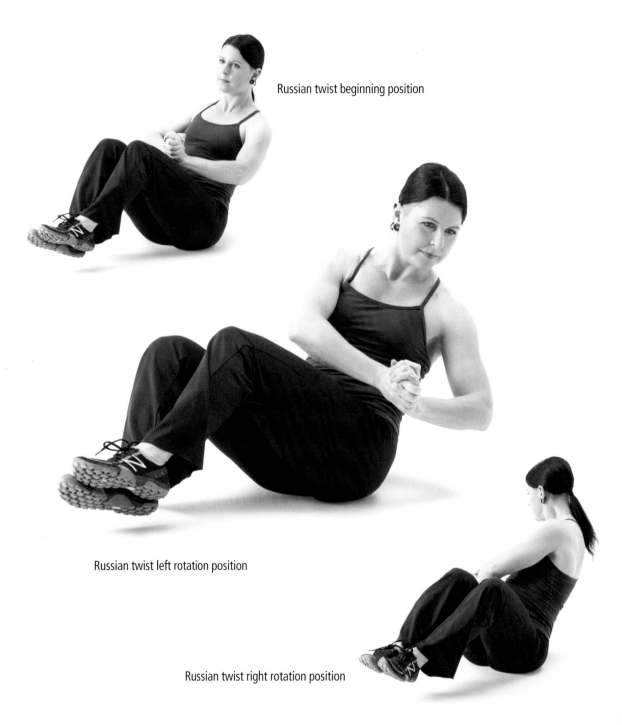

Russian twist beginning position

Russian twist left rotation position

Russian twist right rotation position

## Explosive Fingers

Place both hands out in front of you with your elbows bent. Make a tight fist, then explosively open your fingers. Repeat this movement as rapidly as possible. Continue this exercise for the required amount of time.

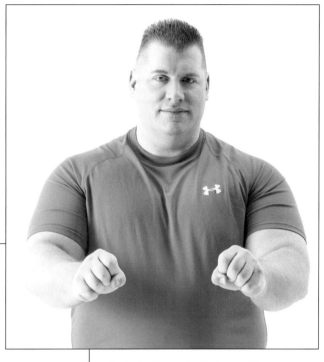

Explosive fingers beginning position

Explosive fingers finish position

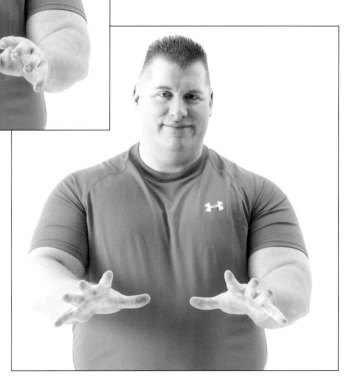

# Bodyweight Isometrics Lower Body

## The Towel Deadlift

This exercise requires the use of a heavy towel. Stand on the middle of the towel with your feet shoulder length apart. Now, squat down and grasp the ends of the towel with the hands. Create tension in the body as you resist against the towel. Power exhale through pursed lips as you hold this isometric contraction for 7 to 12 seconds.

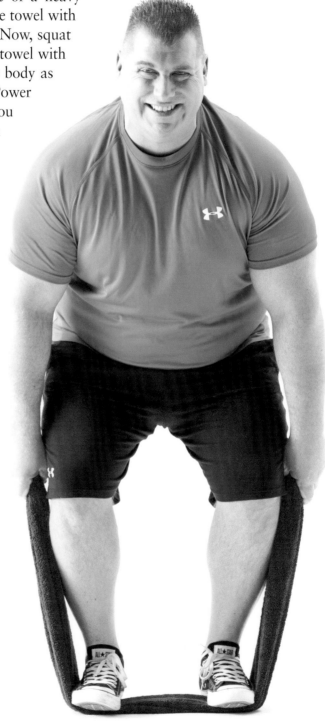

## The Isometric Wall Squat Quadriceps Emphasis

   Begin by standing with your back facing a wall. Now, squat down until your thighs are parallel with the ground and your back is flat against the wall. Using your feet, try to push yourself back through the wall. Gradually increase tension and squeeze the quads while you power exhale through the mouth. Continue this isometric contraction for 7 to 12 seconds.

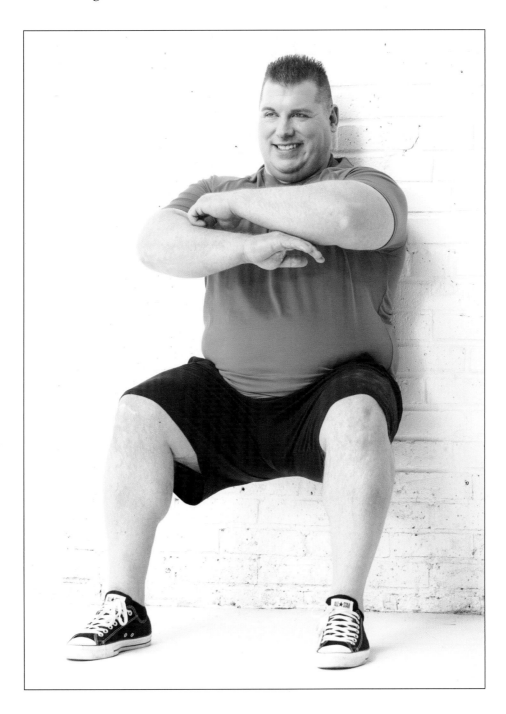

# The Isometric Wall Squat Hamstring Emphasis

With your back facing a wall, squat down until your thighs are parallel with the ground and your back is flat against the wall. Now, drive your heels into the floor trying to pull them into the wall. Gradually increase tension and squeeze the hamstrings while you power exhale through the mouth. Continue this isometric contraction for 7 to 12 seconds.

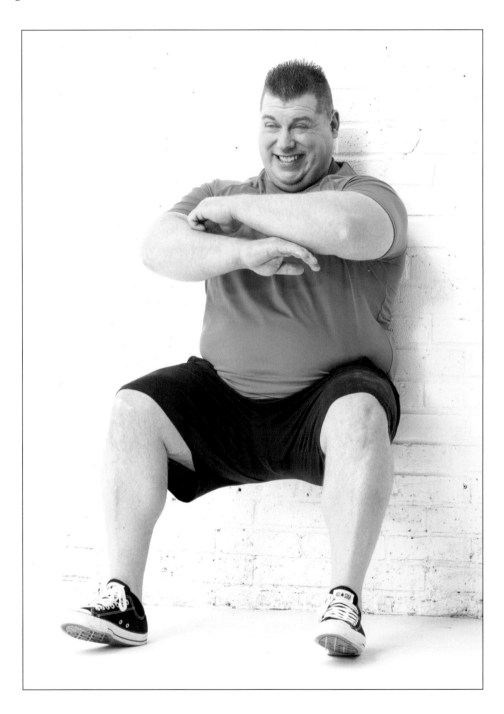

## The Spread the Floor Isometric Squat

With your feet shoulder length apart, squat down until your thighs are parallel with the floor. Now, try to spread the floor with your feet.   Gradually increase tension and squeeze the muscles in your legs as you power exhale through the mouth.   Continue this isometric contraction for 7 to 12 seconds.

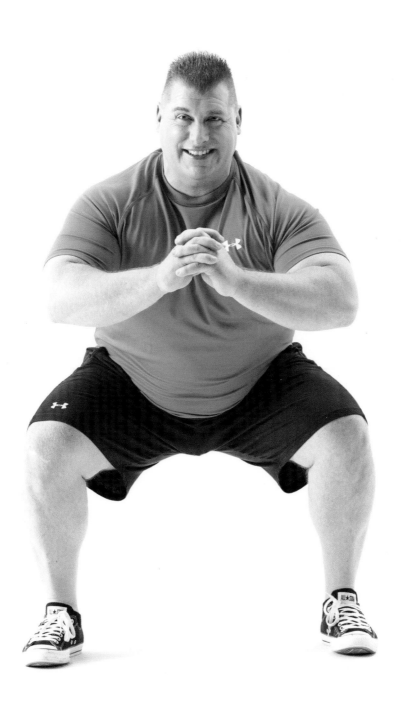

## The Standing Quadriceps Isometric Flex

Begin by standing with your feet shoulder length apart. Now, pull your kneecaps up and squeeze the quadriceps as hard as possible. As you increase the tension, power exhale through the mouth. Continue this isometric flexion for 7 to 12 seconds.

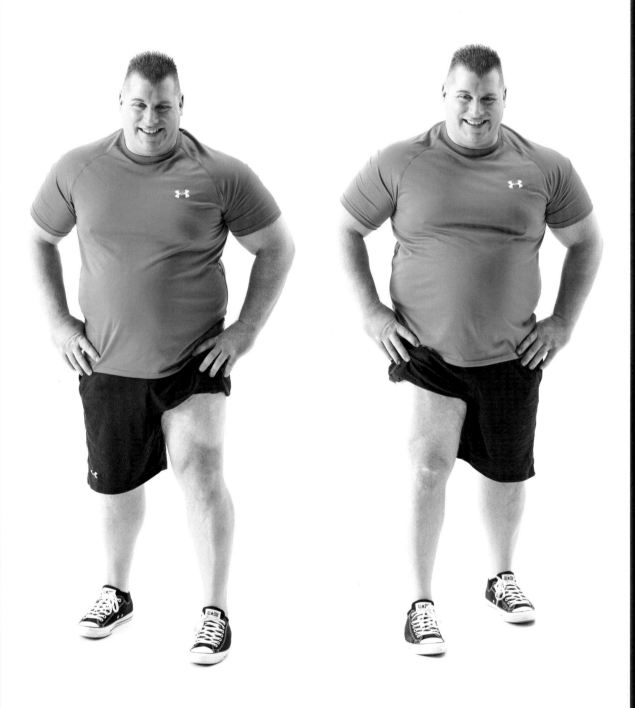

# The Standing Hamstring Isometric Flex

Standing with your feet shoulder length apart, slightly bend one knee and slowly drive your heel toward your glutes. Stop when your foot is around 6 to 12 inches off the ground. In this position, flex the hamstring muscle as hard as possible. As you increase the tension, power exhale through the mouth. Continue this isometric flexion for 7 to 12 seconds. Repeat this exercise on the opposite leg.

## Standing Calf Isometric Flex

Begin by standing with your feet shoulder length apart. Now, bring both heels up off the floor until you feel tension in the calf muscles. Now squeeze the calves as hard as possible. As you increase the tension, power exhale through the mouth. Continue this isometric flexion for 7 to 12 seconds.

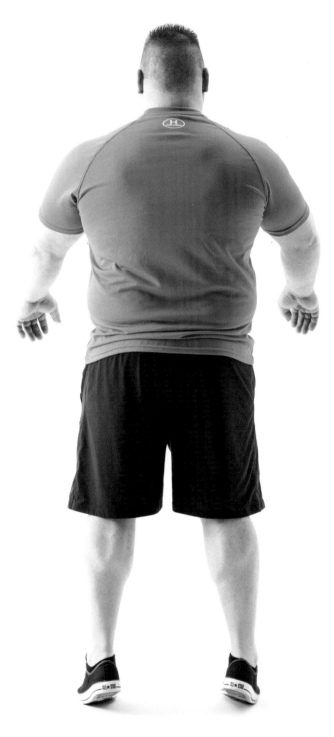

# The Superman Lower Back Isometric Flex

Start by laying on the ground face down with your arms stretched out in front of you. Now, bring your legs and arms off of the floor so that your body is supported by your lower abdomen. Squeeze your lower back muscles hard. As you increase the tension, power exhale through the mouth. Continue this isometric flexion for 7 to 12 seconds.

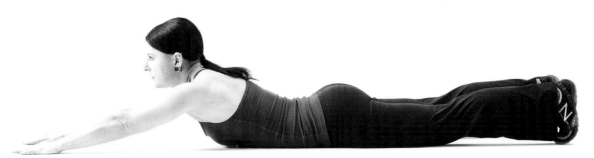

Superman lower back isometric flex beginning

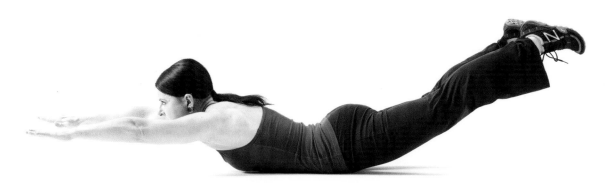

Superman lower back isometric flex finish

# Bodyweight Isometrics Upper Body

## The Crossover Chest Isometric Flex

From a standing position, cross both of your arms in front of your abdominals. Your wrists should be turned so that both thumbs are pointing straight at you. Now, contract your chest muscles as hard as possible. As you increase the tension, power exhale through the mouth. Continue this isometric flexion for 7 to 12 seconds.

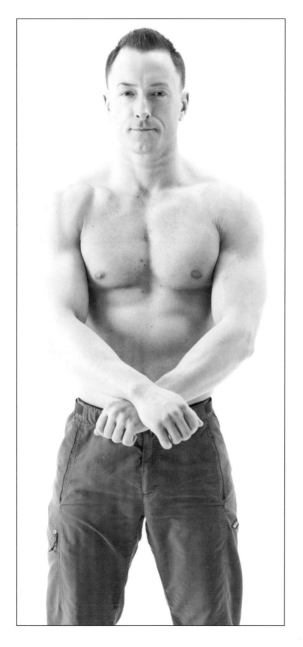
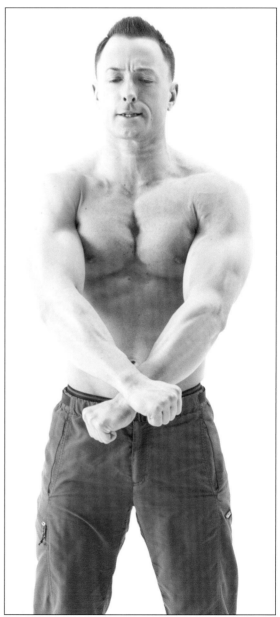

# The Yoga Block Isometric Chest Crush

This exercise requires a standard yoga block. Standing with your feet shoulder width apart, hold a yoga block lengthwise at chest level with your palms. Now, with your elbows slightly bent try to crush the yoga block. As you continue this crushing motion, contract the muscles of the chest as hard as possible. As you increase the tension, power exhale through the mouth. Continue this isometric flexion for 7 to 12 seconds.

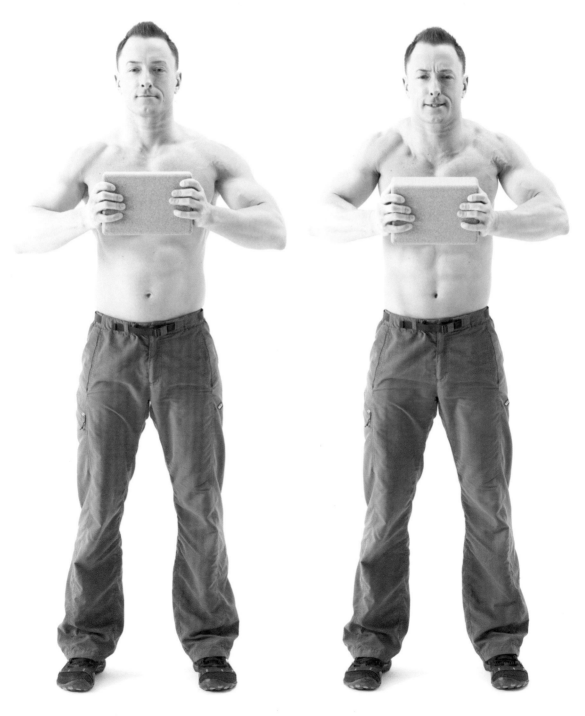

## The Towel Bow Pull

To perform this exercise you will need a heavy duty towel. Begin by grasping the end of the towel with one hand extended straight out to your side. Now, with the other hand grasp the towel at chest level. The position looks like an archer getting ready to pull a bow backward. Try to pull the towel apart. As you continue this pulling motion contract the muscles of the back as hard as possible. As you increase the tension, power exhale through the mouth. Continue this isometric flexion for 7 to 12 seconds. Repeat this exercise in the opposite direction.

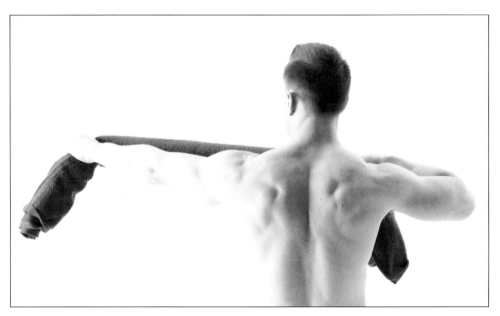

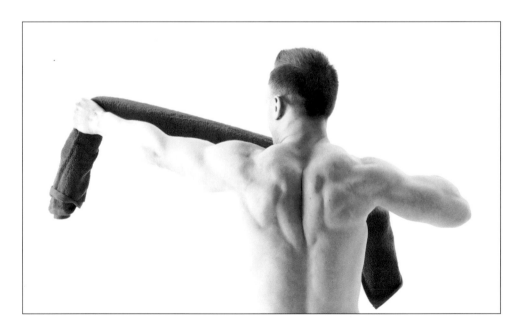

## The Upper Back Isometric Flex

From a standing position, bring your hands behind your head and interlace your fingers. Now, try to pull your hands apart. Contract the lat muscles as hard as possible throughout this exercise. As you increase the tension, power exhale through the mouth. Continue this isometric flexion or 7 to 12 seconds.

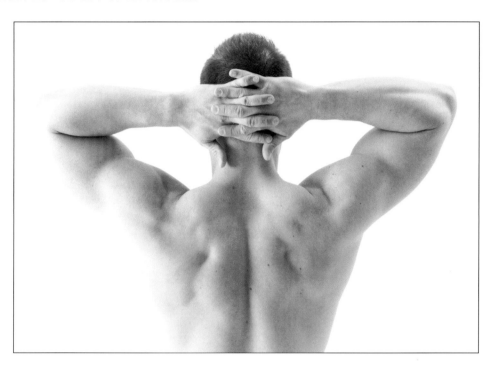

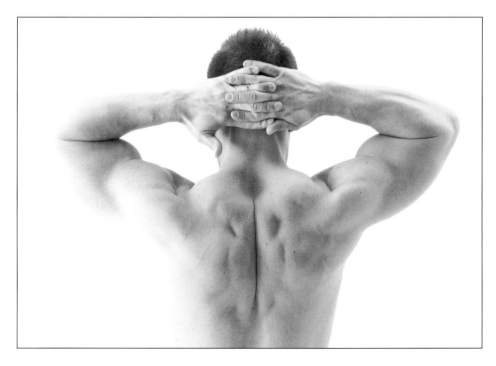

## The Isometric Lat Pull

Find a bar or a high backed chair that is about chest high. With your arms straight in front of you, place both hands on the bar. Now, push downward with your hands as hard as possible. Contract the lat muscles as hard as possible throughout this exercise. As you increase the tension, power exhale through the mouth. Continue this isometric contraction for 7 to 12 seconds.

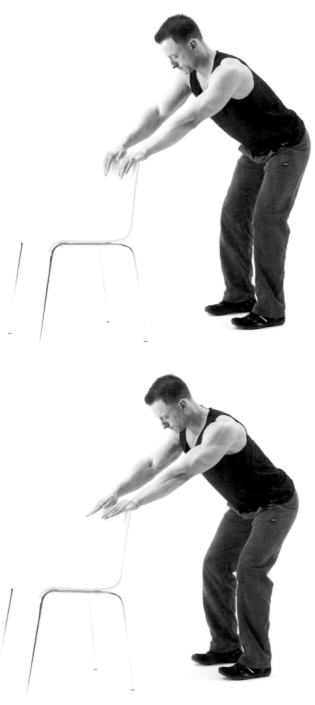

# The Towel Isometric Shoulder Pull

For this exercise you will need a heavy-duty towel. With your hands positioned wider than shoulder width, grasp the towel in an overhand grip. Now, create an intense contraction in the shoulders as you try to pull the towel apart. As you increase the tension, power exhale through the mouth. Continue this isometric contraction for 7 to 12 seconds.

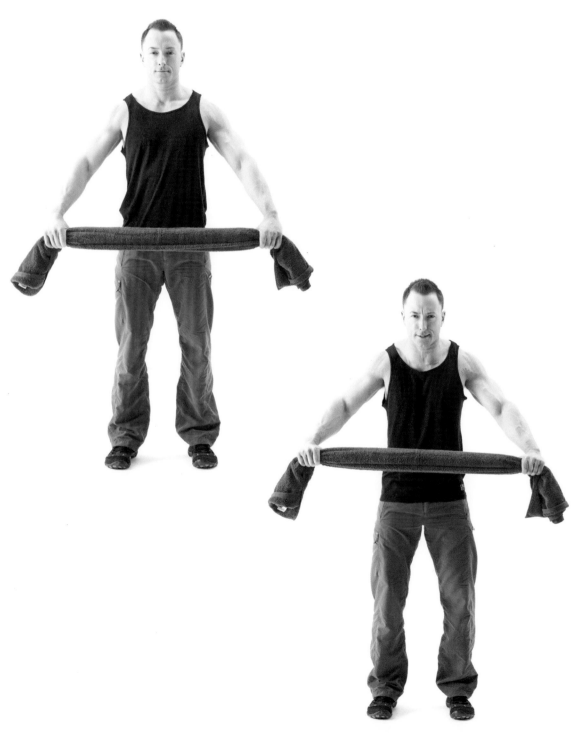

# The Elbow Extension Isometric Shoulder Flex

Bend your elbows and bring your hands to chest level. Now, keeping your arms bent, extend your elbows upward as high as possible. Contract the shoulder muscles as hard as possible throughout this exercise. As you increase the tension, power exhale through the mouth. Continue this isometric flexion for 7 to 12 seconds.

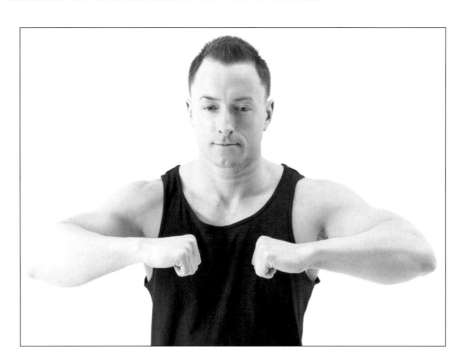

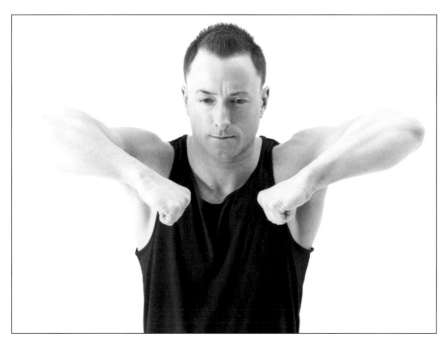

## The Abdominal Isometric Contraction

For this exercise you will need a yoga block or a medicine ball. Lay down on your back with your knees bent and place the yoga block lengthwise in between your knees. Inhale, and slowly bring your shoulders off the ground. Create an intense contraction in the abdominals by squeezing the yoga block and forcing your lower back into the ground. As you increase the tension, power exhale through the mouth. Continue this isometric contraction for 7 to 12 seconds.

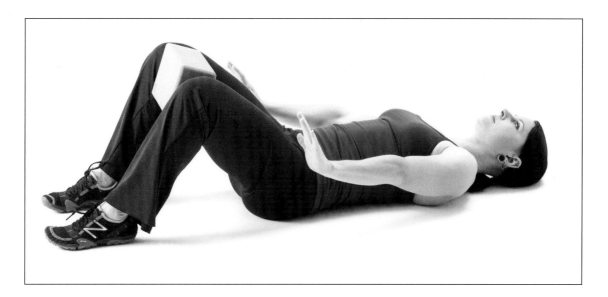

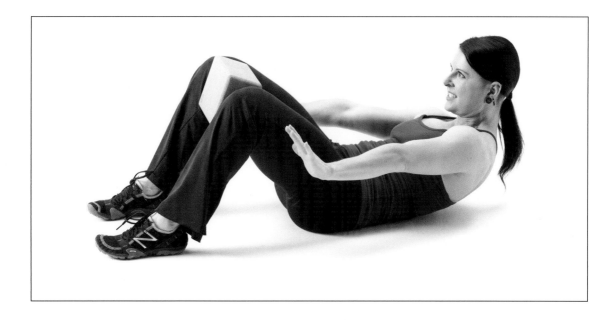

# The Towel Crush

To perform this exercise you will need a heavy towel. From a standing position grasp a rolled up towel with an overhand grip. Crush the towel with your hands as you make a fist. As you increase the tension, power exhale through the mouth. Continue this isometric contraction for 7 to 12 seconds.

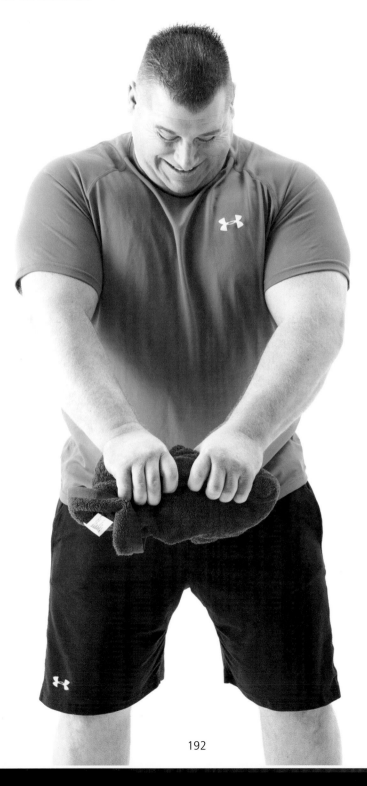

# Neuro-Rack Isometrics

The Neuro-Rack is a piece of equipment that I invented to produce tremendous strength gains. Many people would like to perform heavy-duty isometric exercise, but don't have access to a power rack. The solution is the Neuro-Rack. It is portable, heavy-duty, and accessible. The Neuro-Rack is the perfect companion for champion powerlifters, as well as bodyweight enthusiasts. The Neuro-Rack is a great isometric tool for Neuro-Mass workouts.

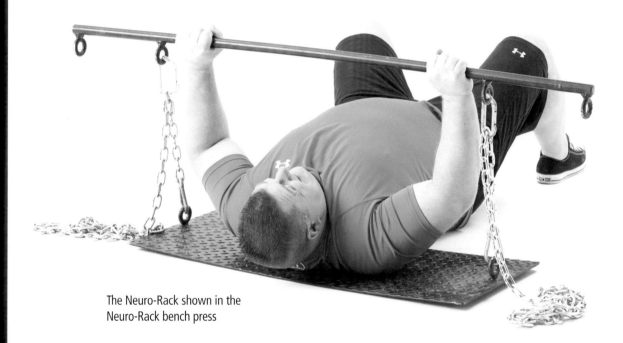

The Neuro-Rack shown in the
Neuro-Rack bench press

## The Neuro-Rack Deadlift

To begin this exercise, set the bar and chains so that they are at knee level. Now, stand on the platform and grasp the bar with an overhand grip. Try to break the chains as you pull straight upward against the immovable resistance. As you gradually increase the tension, power exhale through the mouth. Continue this isometric contraction for 7 to 12 seconds.

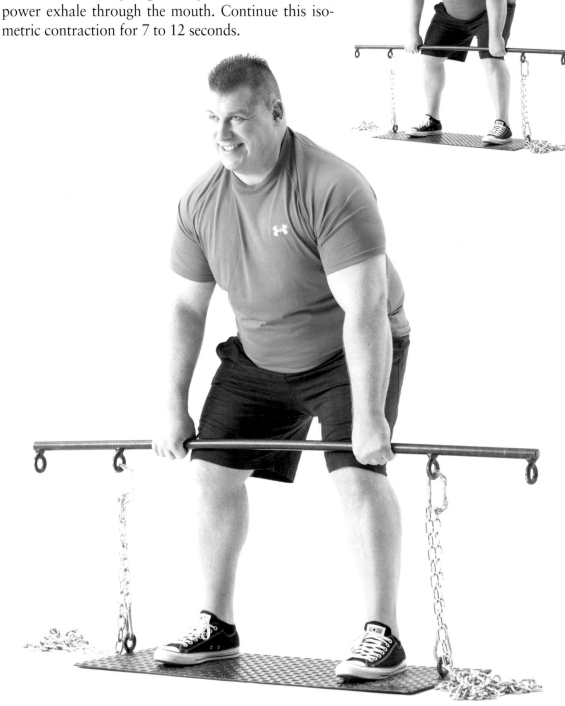

## The Neuro-Rack Squat

Begin by setting the bar and chains to the middle position of the power squat. Step onto the platform and allow the bar to rest on your upper back as you grasp the bar with your hands. Now, try to break the chains as you squat straight up against the immovable resistance. As you gradually increase the tension, power exhale through the mouth. Continue this isometric contraction for 7 to 12 seconds.

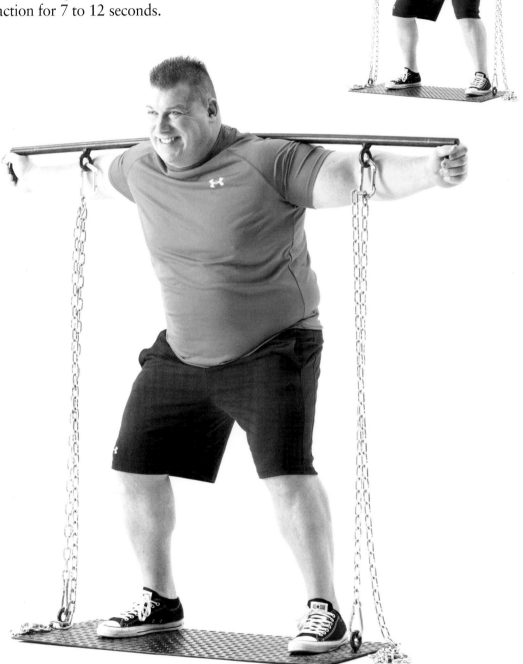

195

## The Neuro-Rack Bench Press

Start by setting the bar and chains to the middle position of a bench press. Lay down with your back flat against the platform. Grasp the bar with a wider than shoulder length grip. Now, try to break the chains as you press straight up against the immovable resistance. As you gradually increase the tension, power exhale through the mouth. Continue this isometric contraction for 7 to 12 seconds.

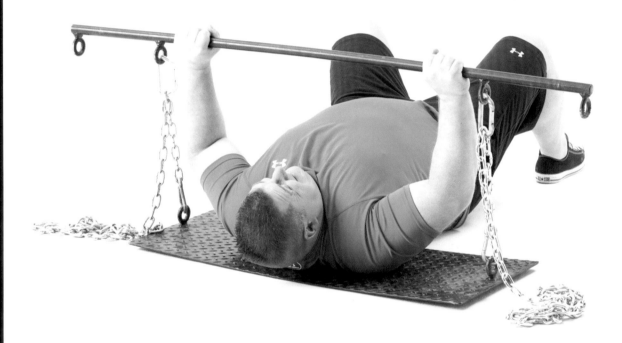

## The Neuro-Rack Overhead Press

To perform this exercise set the bar and chains so that they are just above eye level. Stand on the platform with your feet shoulder length apart. Grasp the bar, and try to break the chains as you press upward against the immovable resistance. As you gradually increase the tension, power exhale through the mouth. Continue this isometric contraction for 7 to 12 seconds.

By incorporating Neuro-Rack isometrics into your Neuro-Mass program, you'll see your strength levels skyrocket.

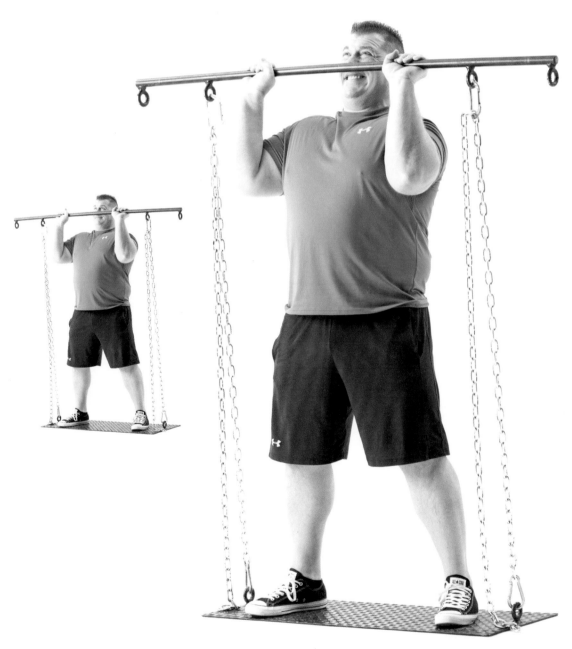

# The Neuro-Burner

Even though it is optional, many athletes will want to incorporate some form of cardio training into the Neuro-Mass program. Long endurance cardio is counterproductive to building smart muscle. I searched for a way that athletes could continue to build mass and still gain all the benefits from intense cardio. Enter the "Neuro-Burner."

The Neuro-Burner not only provides a cardio benefit, but also increases reaction time, speed, and work capacity in minimum time. I have tested the Neuro-Burner on many different athletes from MMA fighters to basketball players. All of them found that Neuro-Burner was one of the most effective forms of intense cardio they had experienced.

The Neuro-Burner is made of a heavy-duty material that creates tremendous resistance when operated properly. This piece of equipment can fit in a gym bag or backpack. It is designed to be used with a partner, but can also be attached to a doorframe or power rack.

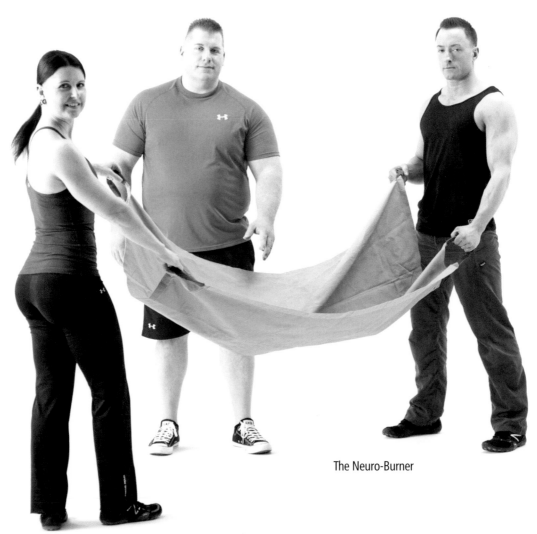

The Neuro-Burner

# The Neuro-Burner Basic Swipe

Grasp the Neuro-Burner by the handles with an overhand grip. Have a partner grasp the other handles or attach them to a doorframe etc. Now, begin to rapidly and explosively snap your arms up and down as the Neuro-Burner resists against the air. Continue this movement for 30 to 60 seconds.

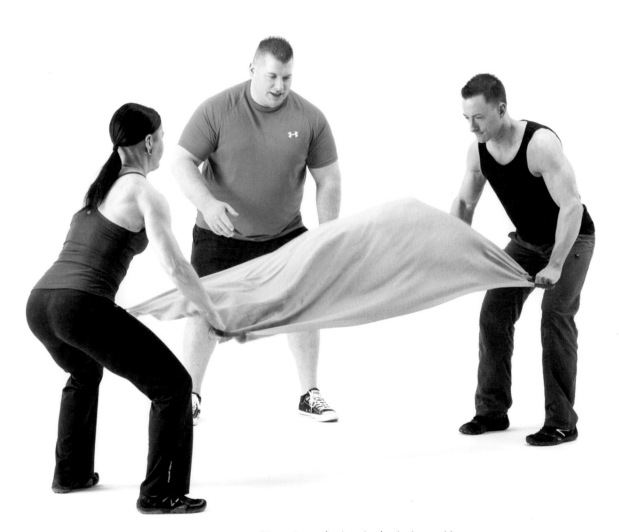

Neuro-Burner basic swipe beginning position

You will find that you are absolutely out of breath and your shoulders are screaming for mercy. There are many more advanced positions and exercises with the Neuro-Burner, but for the purposes of building smart mass, the basic swipe is sufficient.

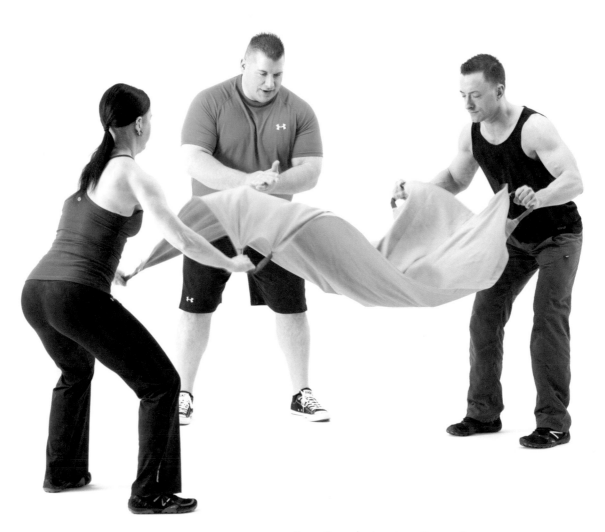

Neuro-Burner basic swipe action position

How to incorporate The Neuro-Burner Swipe into the Neuro-Mass program:

After the completion of your Neuro-Sets, perform three to five rounds of 30 to 60 seconds of the Neuro-Burner basic swipe.

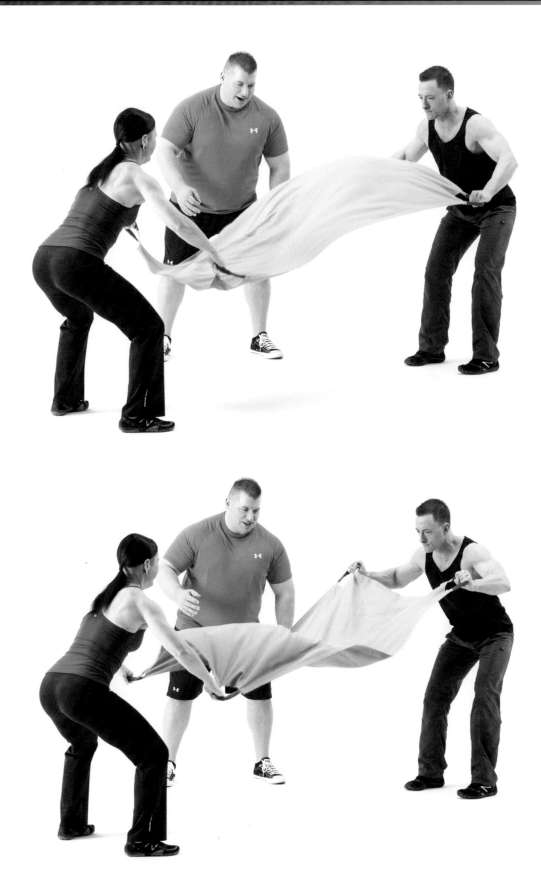

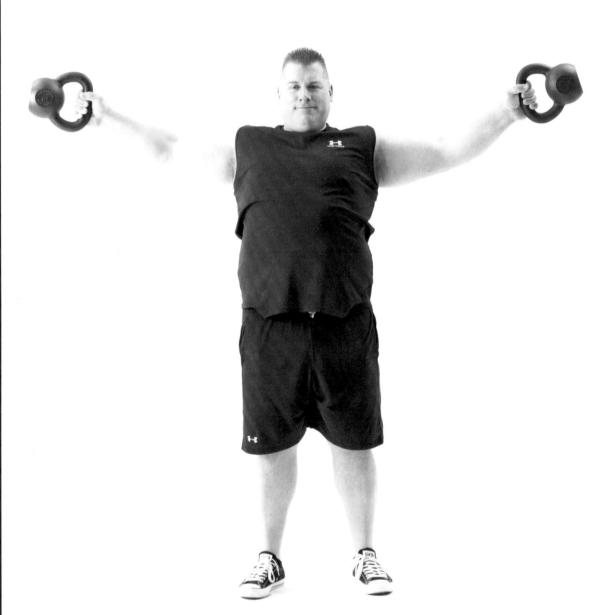

# The Program and Neuro-Sets

*"No citizen has a right to be an amateur in the matter of physical training...what a disgrace it is for a man to grow old without ever seeing the beauty and strength of which his body is capable."*
*– Socrates*

his program is designed for training four days a week. The program can be modified for training three days a week or even two days a week. The key is consistency. Choose the program that best fits you and stick to it. The results will be well worth it.

On training days, you will choose one Neuro-Set for the upper body and one Neuro-Set for the lower body. Perform all the exercises in the Neuro-Set back to back with no break. In between Neuro-Sets you may take a sixty to one hundred twenty second rest. Complete three to five rounds of each Neuro-Set. Make sure to finish all the rounds of one Neuro-Set before moving on to the next. Following the upper body and lower body Neuro-Sets you will perform one Neuro-Set from the supplementary group: the abdominals, grip, or calves. These supplementary Neuro-Sets should be alternated in every workout and should only be performed one time through. Make sure that the same body part emphasis is not trained two days in a row. Optional Neuro-Burner work can also be incorporated three to five times a week.

## Here is a sample of the four day a week program:

Monday-
Lower body quadriceps emphasis Neuro-Set 3-5 times
Upper body chest emphasis Neuro-Set 3-5 times
Abdominals Neuro-Set 1 time
Optional Neuro-Burner work

Tuesday-
Lower body hamstring emphasis Neuro-Set 3-5 times
Upper body shoulder emphasis Neuro-Set 3-5 times
Calves Neuro-Set 1 time

Wednesday- Rest/optional Neuro-Burner work

Thursday-
Lower body quadriceps emphasis Neuro-Set 3-5 times
Upper body back emphasis Neuro-Set 3-5 times
Grip Neuro-Set 1 time

Friday-
Lower body hamstring emphasis Neuro-Set 3-5 times
Upper body chest emphasis Neuro-Set 3-5 times
Abdominals Neuro-Set 1 time
Optional Neuro-Burner work

Saturday-
Rest

Sunday-
Rest

## Sample three day a week program:

Monday-
Lower body quadriceps emphasis Neuro-Set 3-5 times
Upper body chest emphasis Neuro-Set 3-5 times
Abdominals Neuro-Set 1 time
Optional Neuro-Burner work

Tuesday-
Rest

Wednesday- Lower body hamstring emphasis Neuro-Set 3-5 times
Upper body shoulder emphasis Neuro-Set 3-5 times
Calves Neuro-Set 1 time
Optional Neuro-Burner work

Thursday-
Rest

Friday-        Lower body quadriceps emphasis Neuro-Set 3-5 times
               Upper body back emphasis Neuro-Set 3-5
               Grip Neuro-Set 1 time
               Optional Neuro-Burner work

Saturday-      Rest

Sunday-        Rest


## Sample two day a week program:

Monday-        Rest

Tuesday-       Lower body quadriceps emphasis Neuro-Set 3-5 times
               Upper body chest emphasis Neuro-Set 3-5 times
               Abdominals Neuro-Set 1 time
               Optional Neuro-Burner work

Wednesday- Rest

Thursday-      Lower body hamstring emphasis Neuro-Set 3-5 times
               Upper body back emphasis Neuro-Set 3-5 times
               Calves  Neuro-Set 1 time
               Optional Neuro-Burner work

Friday-        Rest

Saturday-      Rest

Sunday-        Rest


With the Neuro-Mass program you will never get bored with workouts again. Also, because of the opportunity for muscle confusion, your gains will never stop. The exciting thing about this program is that the combinations are infinite. For example, on Monday you could do kettlebell Neuro-Sets and Tuesday bodyweight Neuro-Sets.  You can also incorporate hybrid Neuro-Sets at any point in the program. You can also alternate between bodyweight and kettlebell Neuro-Sets in the same workout. To increase intensity, you can choose to add more Neuro-Sets, increase the kettlebell weight, or choose a more difficult Neuro-Set. Neuro-Mass is the ultimate in flexibility and results.

# *Kettlebell Neuro-Sets Quadriceps Emphasis*

1. Double kettlebell front squat – 8 to 12 repetitions
   Single kettlebell explosive lunge – 15 to 60 seconds
   Double kettlebell isometric wall squat quadriceps emphasis – 7 to 12 seconds

2. Double kettlebell lateral step squat – 8 to 12 repetitions
   Kettlebell lateral shuffle –15 to 60 seconds
   Double kettlebell spread the floor isometric squat – 7 to 12 seconds

3. Double kettlebell front elevation lunge – 8 to 12 repetitions
   Double kettlebell high pull to catch squat – 15 to 60 seconds
   Double kettlebell isometric wall squat quadriceps emphasis – 7 to 12 seconds

4. Double kettlebell rear elevation lunge – 8 to 12 repetitions
   Double kettlebell outside the legs swing – 15 to 60 seconds
   Double kettlebell isometric wall squat quadriceps emphasis – 7 to 12 seconds

5. Double kettlebell wide squats – 8 to 12 repetitions
   Single kettlebell jump squats – 15 to 60 seconds
   Double kettlebell isometric wall squat quadriceps emphasis – 7 to 12 seconds

6. Double kettlebell ballet squats – 8 to 12 repetitions
   Double kettlebell jump squats – 15 to 60 seconds
   Double kettlebell isometric wall squat quadriceps emphasis – 7 to 12 seconds

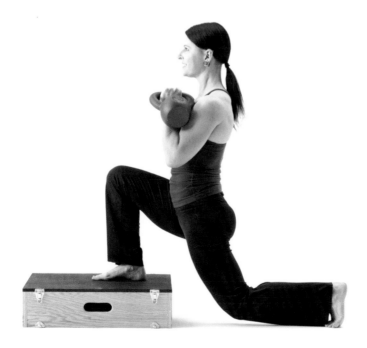

# Kettlebell Neuro-Sets Hamstring Emphasis

1. Double kettlebell sumo deadlift – 8 to 12 repetitions
   Double kettlebell mule kick combo – 15 to 60 seconds
   Double kettlebell isometric wall squat hamstring emphasis – 7 to 12 seconds

2. Double kettlebell suitcase deadlift – 8 to 12 repetitions
   Single kettlebell anchor sprints – 15 to 60 seconds
   Double kettlebell isometric wall squats hamstring emphasis – 7 to 12 seconds

3. Double kettlebell sumo deadlift – 8 to 12 repetitions
   Single kettlebell walking swing – 15 to 60 seconds
   Double kettlebell isometric wall squat hamstring emphasis – 7 to 12 seconds

4. Double kettlebell suitcase deadlift – 8 to 12 repetitions
   Kettlebell reverse hyperextension – 15 to 60 seconds
   Kettlebell isometric wall squat hamstring emphasis – 7 to 12 seconds

5. Double kettlebell sumo deadlift – 8 to 12 repetitions
   Single kettlebell anchor sprints – 15 to 60 seconds
   Kettlebell hyperextension isometric contraction – 7 to 12 seconds

6. Double kettlebell suitcase deadlift – 8 to 12 repetitions
   Double kettlebell mule kick combo – 15 to 60 seconds
   Double kettlebell isometric wall squat hamstring emphasis – 7 to 12 seconds

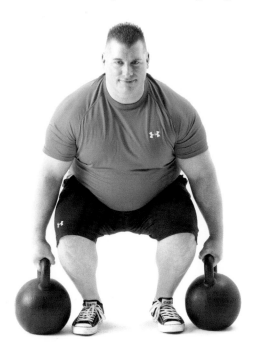

# *Kettlebell Neuro-Sets Chest Emphasis*

1. Double kettlebell bench press – 8 to 12 repetitions
   Double kettlebell rolling speed press – 15 to 60 seconds
   Kettlebell chest crush isometric – 7 to 12 seconds

2. Double kettlebell incline bench press – 8 to 12 repetitions
   Kettlebell primal shakers standing position – 15 to 60 seconds
   Upside down kettlebell chest crush isometric plank position – 7 to 12 seconds

3. Double kettlebell bench flyes – 8 to 12 repetitions
   Kettlebell primal shakers sit up position – 15 to 60 seconds
   Kettlebell chest crush isometric – 7 to 12 seconds

4. Kettlebell crush press – 8 to 12 repetitions
   Double kettlebell rolling speed press – 15 to 60 seconds
   Kettlebell chest crush isometric – 7 to 12 seconds

5. Kettlebell bench press – 8 to 12 repetitions
   Kettlebell primal shakers standing position – 15 to 60 seconds
   Upside down kettlebell chest crush isometric plank position – 7 to 12 seconds

6. Double kettlebell incline bench press – 8 to 12 repetitions
   Kettlebell primal shakers sit up position – 15 to 60 seconds
   Kettlebell chest crushed isometric – 7 to 12 seconds

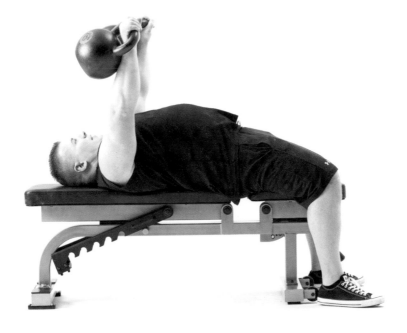

# Kettlebell Neuro-Sets Shoulder Emphasis

1. Double kettlebell overhead press – 8 to 12 repetitions
   Double kettlebell speed see saw press – 15 to 60 seconds
   Double kettlebell isometric lateral raise – 7 to 12 seconds

2. Double kettlebell bottoms up overhead press – 8 to 12 repetitions
   Kettlebell high pull from squat – 15 to 60 seconds
   Kettlebell isometric chest pull – 7 to 12 seconds

3. Double kettlebell crucifix – 8 to 12 repetitions
   Kettlebell front raise snatch – 15 to 60 seconds
   Kettlebell isometric shoulder press – 7 to 12 seconds

4. Double kettlebell overhead press – 8 to 12 repetitions
   Double kettlebell hang cleans – 15 to 60 seconds
   Kettlebell isometric shoulder press – 7 to 12 seconds

5. Double kettlebell bottoms up overhead press – 8 to 12 repetitions
   Double kettlebell front raise snatch – 15 to 60 seconds
   Double kettlebell isometric lateral raise – 7 to 12 seconds

6. Double kettlebell crucifix –
   8 to 12 repetitions

   Double kettlebell see saw
   press – 15 to 60 seconds

   Double kettlebell isometric
   lateral raise – 7 to 12 seconds

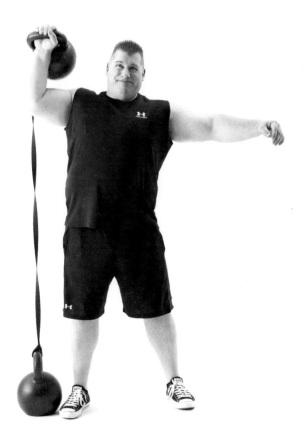

# *Kettlebell Neuro-Sets Back Emphasis*

1. Double kettlebell bent over row – 8 to 12 repetitions
   Double kettlebell bear crawl – 15 to 60 seconds
   Double kettlebell isometric row – 7 to 12 seconds

2. Kettlebell crush inverted row – 8 to 12 repetitions
   Double kettlebell speed row – 15 to 60 seconds
   Double kettlebell isometric row – 7 to 12 seconds

3. Kettlebell crush pull up – 8 to 12 repetitions
   Kettlebell cross body snatch – 15 to 60 seconds
   Kettlebell isometric pull up – 7 to 12 seconds

4. Double kettlebell bent over row – 8 to 12 repetitions
   Double kettlebell speed row – 15 to 60 seconds
   Double kettlebell isometric row – 7 to 12 seconds

5. Kettlebell crush pull up – 8 to 12 repetitions
   Double kettlebell bear crawl – 15 to 60 seconds
   Double kettlebell isometric row – 7 to 12 seconds

6. Kettlebell crush inverted row – 8 to 12 repetitions
   Kettlebell cross body snatch – 15 to 60 seconds
   Kettlebell isometric pull up – 7 to 12 seconds

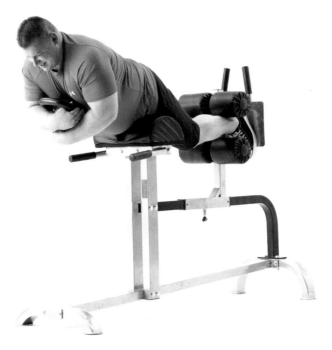

# Supplementary Kettlebell Neuro-Sets

## *Kettlebell Neuro-Set Abdominal Emphasis*

Standing double kettlebell twist – 8 to 12 repetitions
Kettlebell seated twist – 15 to 60 seconds
Kettlebell isometric crunch – 7 to 12 seconds

## *Kettlebell Neuro-Sets Calf Emphasis*

1. Double kettlebell calf raise – 8 to 12 repetitions
   Double kettlebell calf jumps – 15 to 60 seconds
   Double kettlebell calf raise isometric contraction – 7 to 12 seconds

2. Double kettlebell calf raise – 8 to 12 repetitions
   Double kettlebell toe curl – 15 to 60 seconds
   Double kettlebell calf raise isometric contraction – 7 to 12 seconds

## *Kettlebell Neuro-Set Grip Emphasis*

Kettlebell claw curl – 8 to 12 repetitions
Kettlebell hand-to-hand swings – 15 to 60 seconds
Kettlebell towel crush – 7 to 12 seconds

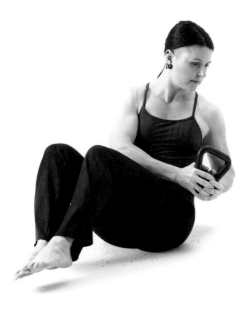

# Bodyweight Neuro-Sets

## *Bodyweight Neuro-Sets Quadriceps Emphasis*

1. Regular squats – 8 to 12 repetitions
   Explosive lunges – 15 to 60 seconds
   Isometric wall squats quadriceps emphasis – 7 to 12 seconds

2. Ballet squats – 8 to 12 repetitions
   Jump squats – 15 to 60 seconds
   Standing quadriceps isometric flexion – 7 to 12 seconds

3. Front elevation lunge – 8 to 12 repetitions
   Broad jump – 15 to 60 seconds
   Isometric wall squat quadriceps emphasis – 7 to 12 seconds

4. Rear elevation lunge – 8 to 12 repetitions
   Platform jump – 15 to 60 seconds
   Isometric wall squat quadriceps emphasis – 7 to 12 seconds

5. Wide squats – 8 to 12 repetitions

   Lateral shuffle – 15 to 60 seconds

   Spread the floor isometric squat –
   7 to 12 seconds

6. Lateral step squat –
   8 to 12 repetitions

   Lateral hops – 15 to 60 seconds

   Spread the floor isometric squat –
   7 to 12 seconds

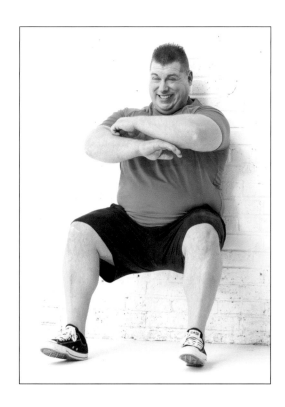

# *Bodyweight Neuro-Set Hamstring Emphasis*

1. Romanian deadlift – 8 to 12 repetitions
   Anchor sprints – 15 to 60 seconds
   Towel deadlift – 7 to 12 seconds

2. Single leg deadlift – 8 to 12 repetitions
   Mule kicks – 15 to 60 seconds
   Standing hamstring isometric flexion – 7 to 12 seconds

3. Glute ham raise – 8 to 12 repetitions
   Hanging lower body catch and throw – 15 to 60 seconds
   Isometric wall squat hamstring emphasis – 7 to 12 seconds

4. Romanian deadlift – 8 to 12 repetitions
   Bootstrappers – 15 to 60 seconds
   Towel deadlift – 7 to 12 seconds

5. Glute ham raise – 8 to 12 repetitions
   Bodyweight reverse hyperextensions – 15 to 60 seconds
   Superman lower back isometric flexion – 7 to 12 seconds

6. Single leg deadlift –
   8 to 12 repetitions

   Arms overhead anchor sprints –
   15 to 60 seconds

   Isometric wall squat hamstring
   emphasis – 7 to 12 seconds

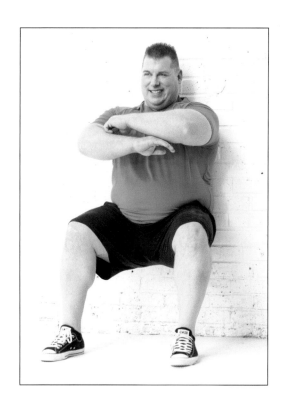

# *Bodyweight Neuro-Sets Chest Emphasis*

1. Neuro-Grip push-ups – 8 to 12 repetitions
   Double strike push-ups – 15 to 60 seconds
   Crossover chest isometric flexion – 7 to 12 seconds

2. Incline wall push-ups – 8 to 12 repetitions
   Floor fire push-ups – 15 to 60 seconds
   Yoga block isometric chest crush – 7 to 12 seconds

3. Sledgehammer push-ups – 8 to 12 repetitions
   Medicine ball bouncing push-ups – 15 to 60 seconds
   Crossover chest isometric flexion – 7 to 12 seconds

4. Chest elevated push-ups – 8 to 12 repetitions
   Heavy bag speed punches – 15 to 60 seconds
   Yoga block isometric chest crush – 7 to 12 seconds

5. Medicine ball crush push-ups – 8 to 12 repetitions
   Lateral moving step push-ups – 15 to 60 seconds
   Crossover chest isometric flexion – 7 to 12 seconds

6. One arm supported push-ups – 8 to 12 repetitions
   Double strike push-ups – 15 to 60 seconds
   Yoga block isometric chest crush – 7 to 12 seconds

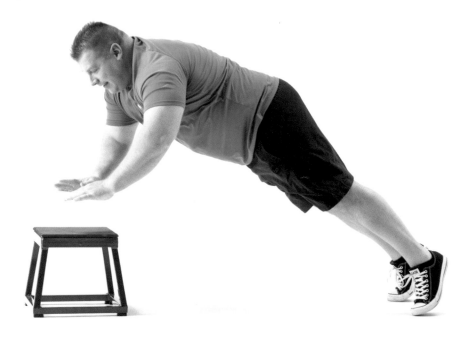

# Bodyweight Neuro-Sets Shoulder Emphasis

1.   Handstand push-ups – 8 to 12 repetitions
     Hummingbird – 15 to 60 seconds
     Towel isometric shoulder pull – 7 to 12 seconds


2.   Shoulder levers – 8 to 12 repetitions
     Hummingbird – 15 to 60 seconds
     Elbow extension isometric shoulder flexion – 7 to 12 seconds


3.   Handstand push-ups – 8 to 12 repetitions
     Seated arms sprints – 15 to 60 seconds
     Towel isometric shoulder pull – 7 to 12 seconds


4.   Shoulder levers – 8 to 12 repetitions
     Seated arms sprints – 15 to 60 seconds
     Towel isometric shoulder pull – 7 to 12 seconds

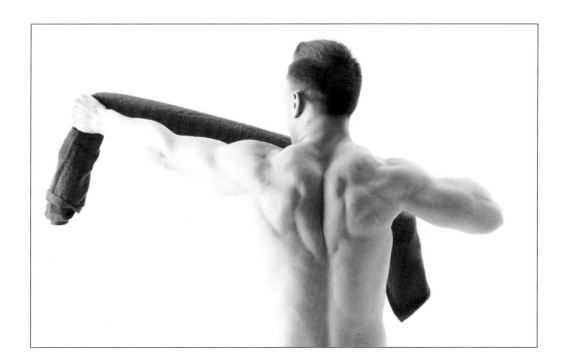

# Bodyweight Neuro-Sets Back Emphasis

1.  Inverted bodyweight row – 8 to 12 repetitions
    Treadmill hand crawl – 15 to 60 seconds
    Towel bow pull – 7 to 12 seconds

2.  Pull-ups – 8 to 12 repetitions
    Pull-up bar walk – 15 to 60 seconds
    Isometric lat pull – 7 to 12 seconds

3.  Pull-ups – 8 to 12 repetitions
    Inverted speed row – 15 to 60 seconds
    Upper back isometric flexion – 7 to 12 seconds

4.  Inverted bodyweight row – 8 to 12 repetitions
    Single leg shoulder bridge – 15 to 60 seconds
    Towel bow pull – 7 to 12 seconds

5.  Pull-ups – 8 to 12 repetitions
    Treadmill hand crawl – 15 to 60 seconds
    Towel bow pull – 7 to 12 seconds

6.  Inverted bodyweight row – 8 to 12 repetitions
    Pull-up bar walk – 15 to 60 seconds
    Isometric lat pull – 7 to 12 seconds

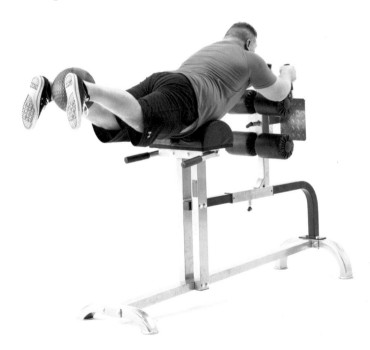

# Bodyweight Supplementary Neuro-Sets

## Bodyweight Neuro-Set Abdominal Emphasis

Hanging leg raise – 8 to 12 repetitions
Russian twists – 15 to 60 seconds
Abdominal isometric contraction – 7 to 12 seconds

## Bodyweight Neuro-Set Calf Emphasis

Single leg calf raise – 8 to 12 repetitions
Wall hops – 15 to 60 seconds
Standing calf isometric flexion – 7 to 12 seconds

## Bodyweight Neuro-Set Grip Emphasis

Inverted bodyweight row claw curl – 8 to 12 repetitions
Explosive fingers – 15 to 60 seconds
Towel crush – 7 to 12 seconds

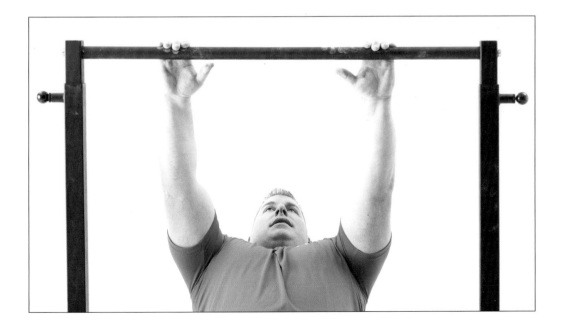

# Hybrid Neuro-Sets Including Kettlebells, Bodyweight, and Neuro-Rack Exercises

## *Hybrid Neuro-Sets Quadriceps Emphasis*

1. Double kettlebell front squat – 8 to 12 repetitions
   Explosive lunges – 15 to 60 seconds
   Neuro-Rack isometric squat – 7 to 12 seconds

2. Double kettlebell front elevation lunge – 8 to 12 repetitions
   Platform jump – 15 to 60 seconds
   Neuro-Rack isometric squat – 7 to 12 seconds

3. Double kettlebell ballet squat – 8 to 12 repetitions
   Jump squats – 15 to 60 seconds
   Neuro-Rack isometric squat – 7 to 12 seconds

4. Double kettlebell lateral step squat – 8 to 12 repetitions
   Lateral hops – 15 to 60 seconds
   Spread the floor isometric squat – 7 to 12 seconds

5. Wide squats – 8 to 12 repetitions
   Single kettlebell jump squats – 15 to 60 seconds
   Isometric wall squat quadriceps emphasis – 7 to 12 seconds

6. Front elevation lunge – 8 to 12 repetitions
   Double kettlebell high pull to catch squat – 15 to 60 seconds
   Standing quadriceps isometric flexion – 7 to 12 seconds

# Hybrid Neuro-Sets Hamstring Emphasis

1. Romanian deadlift – 8 to 12 repetitions
   Double kettlebell mule kick combo – 15 to 60 seconds
   Neuro-Rack isometric deadlift – 7 to 12 seconds

2. Single leg deadlift – 8 to 12 repetitions
   Kettlebell reverse hyperextensions – 15 to 60 seconds
   Neuro-Rack isometric deadlift – 7 to 12 seconds

3. Double kettlebell sumo deadlift – 8 to 12 repetitions
   Bootstrappers – 15 to 60 seconds
   Neuro-Rack isometric deadlift – 7 to 12 seconds

4. Glute ham raise – 8 to 12 repetitions
   Single kettlebell walking swing – 15 to 60 seconds
   Neuro-Rack isometric deadlift – 7 to 12 seconds

5. Double kettlebell sumo deadlift – 8 to 12 repetitions
   Hanging lower body catch and throw – 15 to 60 seconds
   Double kettlebell isometric wall squat hamstring emphasis – 7 to 12 seconds

6. Romanian deadlift – 8 to 12 repetitions
   Single kettlebell anchor sprints – 15 to 60 seconds
   Isometric wall squat hamstring emphasis – 7 to 12 seconds

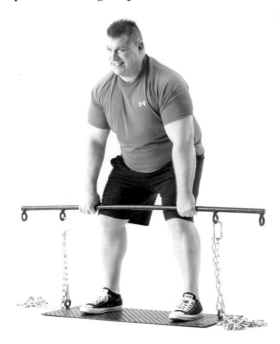

# Hybrid Neuro-Sets Chest Emphasis

1.  Neuro-Grip push-ups – 8 to 12 repetitions
    Double kettlebell rolling speed press – 15 to 60 seconds
    Neuro-Rack isometric benchpress – 7 to 12 seconds

2.  Incline wall push-ups – 8 to 12 repetitions
    Kettlebell primal shakers – 15 to 60 seconds
    Neuro-Rack isometric benchpress – 7 to 12 seconds

3.  Sledgehammer push-ups – 8 to 12 repetitions
    Double kettlebell rolling speed press – 15 to 60 seconds
    Neuro-Rack isometric benchpress – 7 to 12 seconds

4.  Double kettlebell benchpress – 8 to 12 repetitions
    Double strike push-ups – 15 to 60 seconds
    Neuro-Rack isometric benchpress – 7 to 12 seconds

5.  Double kettlebell bench flyes – 8 to 12 repetitions
    Heavy bag speed punches – 15 to 60 seconds
    Yoga block isometric chest crush – 7 to 12 seconds

6.  Kettlebell crush press – 8 to 12 repetitions
    Medicine ball bouncing push-ups – 15 to 60 seconds
    Crossover chest isometric flexion – 7 to 12 seconds

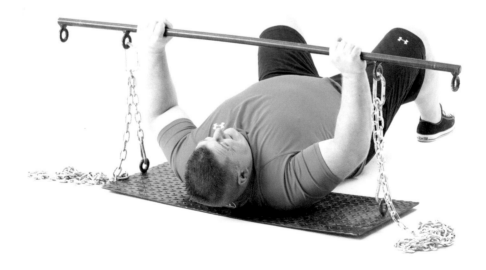

# Hybrid Neuro-Sets Shoulder Emphasis

1. Double kettlebell overhead press – 8 to 12 repetitions
   Hummingbird – 15 to 60 seconds
   Neuro-Rack isometric overhead press – 7 to 12 seconds

2. Handstand push-ups – 8 to 12 repetitions
   Kettlebell front raise snatch – 15 to 60 seconds
   Neuro-Rack isometric overhead press – 7 to 12 seconds

3. Shoulder levers – 8 to 12 repetitions
   Double kettlebell see saw press – 15 to 60 seconds
   Neuro-Rack isometric overhead press – 7 to 12 seconds

4. Double kettlebell bottoms up overhead press – 8 to 12 repetitions
   Hummingbird – 15 to 60 seconds
   Neuro-Rack isometric overhead press – 7 to 12 seconds

5. Double kettlebell crucifix – 8 to 12 repetitions
   Seated arms sprints – 15 to 60 seconds
   Towel isometric shoulder pull – 7 to 12 seconds

6. Handstand push-ups – 8 to 12 repetitions
   Double kettlebell hang cleans – 15 to 60 seconds
   Elbow extension isometric shoulder flexion – 7 to 12 seconds

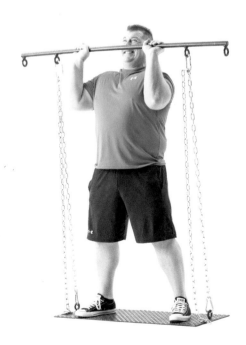

# *Hybrid Neuro-Sets Back Emphasis*

1. Double kettlebell bent over row – 8 to 12 repetitions
   Inverted speed row – 15 to 60 seconds
   Double kettlebell isometric row – 7 to 12 seconds

2. Pull-ups – 8 to 12 repetitions
   Kettlebell cross body snatch – 15 to 60 seconds
   Upper back isometric flexion – 7 to 12 seconds

3. Inverted bodyweight row – 8 to 12 repetitions
   Double kettlebell speed row – 15 to 60 seconds
   Towel bow pull – 7 to 12 seconds

4. Kettlebell crush pull-up – 8 to 12 repetitions
   Pull-up bar walk – 15 to 60 seconds
   Towel bow pull – 7 to 12 seconds

5. Inverted bodyweight row – 8 to 12 repetitions
   Double kettlebell bear crawl – 15 to 60 seconds
   Isometric lat pull – 7 to 12 seconds

6. Double kettlebell bent over row –
   8 to 12 repetitions

   Pull-up bar walk –
   15 to 60 seconds

   Upper back isometric flexion –
   7 to 12 seconds

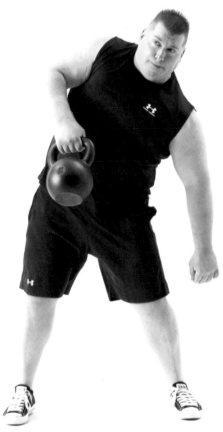

# Neuro-Focus

"In the sports arena I would say there is nothing
like training and preparation.
You have to train your mind as much as your body."
–Venus Williams

**N**euro-Mass workouts require that you be "all in". The Neuro-Sets will demand total focus, concentration, and great physical effort. To get the most out of this program you will not be able to just go through the motions. The body does not enjoy discipline. Therefore, we often procrastinate in doing workouts. Another key issue during exercise is lack of focus, allowing the mind to drift during workouts. The solution to these problems is "Neuro-Focus."

Neuro-Focus exercises will focus your mind, develop your willpower, and deepen your concentration skills. This is accomplished by stimulating the prefrontal cortex. I understand the importance of focus every time I break a stack of bricks, or drive a nail through board with my hand. Without proper focus and concentration, I would not be able to accomplish the feats of strength that I do in my programs. By taking just a few minutes to do this mental warm-up, you'll take your Neuro-Mass workouts to a whole new level.

## Numbers Quick Count

Count out loud from 0 to 150 as quickly as possible. This type of rapid out loud counting has been shown to increase activity and blood flow in the prefrontal cortex. It is also a great way to clear your mind, as you prepare to focus on your workout.

## Words Quick Count

Start by picking a page out of a book, magazine, or newspaper. Now, count out loud every word on the page as fast as you can, starting from the top. To increase the difficulty start counting from the bottom and work your way to the top.

## Reading Out Loud

Pick a passage from a book and read it out loud. The prefrontal cortex is stimulated most when the reading is done with great expression.

## Juggling

Pick up three beanbags or balls and perform basic juggling. This kind of exercise used as a warm-up really increases the mind and body connection. You may also choose to juggle a light kettlebell, performing various flips and tosses.

## Body Awareness

Take a moment and close your eyes. Now, begin to mentally ask yourself the following questions. What do I hear? What temperature is my body? Am I feeling tight or loose? How is my breathing? Taking time to ask those questions tunes you into your body and creates the proper focus for training.

## Goal Concentration

Find an object or word that best describes your goal for the workout. Focus your eyes and mind on the word or object for 2 to 3 min. During this time of concentration practice slow abdominal breathing. This simple exercise helps our mind to take a break from processing all the daily external information, and helps us to focus on our goal.

Simply choose two or three of the Neuro-Focus exercises and perform them prior to your workout. The whole process should not take longer than 5-7 minutes.

# Preparing the Nervous System For Action with the Neuro-Strike and the Neuro-Stomp

There are many excellent ways to warm up the body and prepare it for exercise. These include dynamic stretching and mobility drills. One of the most overlooked ways to prepare for athletic pursuits is the use of controlled striking and stomping. The Neuro-Strike will wake up the nervous system, stimulate the release of lymphatic fluid, increase energy and workout intensity.

## Neuro-Strike Techniques

### Slapping

This involves the use of your fingers to gently slap your body. Start by gently slapping your upper body beginning with the arms and moving all the way down to the legs.

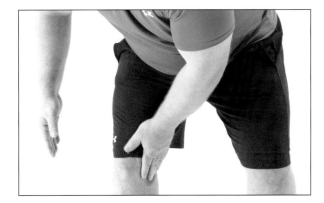

Slapping stimulates nerve endings, as well as prepares the body to absorb impact.

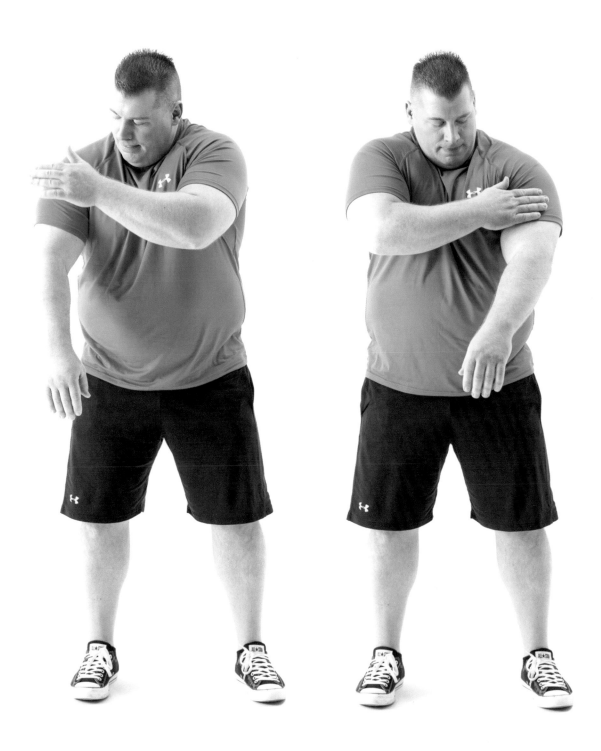

# Hacking

This technique utilizes the outer edge of the hand, sometimes referred to as a "knife edge" in some martial arts circles.  Hacking is used to break up tight knotted up muscles, and improve blood flow.  This hacking motion should be very light starting with the upper body and moving throughout the lower body. The chopping motion should not be too hard, this is not Ric Flair performing knife edge chops on someone's chest.

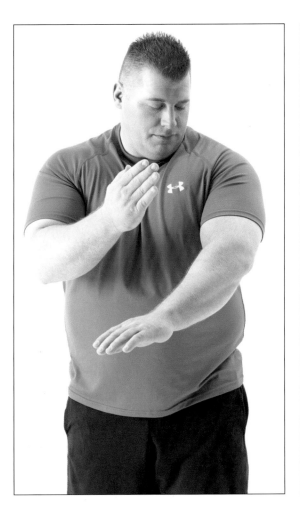 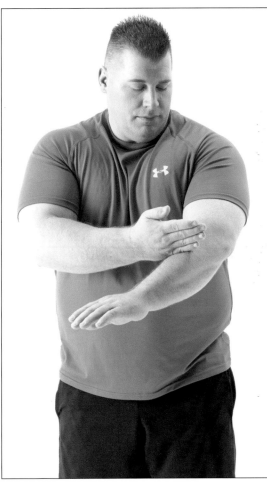

# Tapping

Tapping involves using your fingertips only to lightly tap the muscles and pressure points to awaken the nervous system. Begin by working through the upper body and continue to move on down to the lower body. This technique will increase blood flow, energy and body awareness.

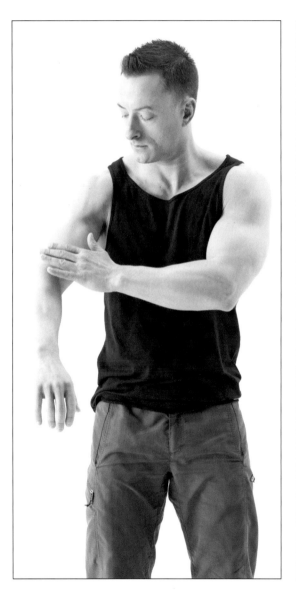
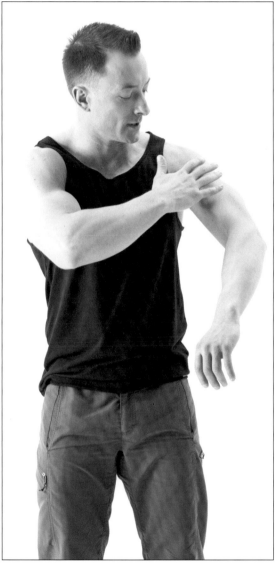

# Cupping

This technique involves using your hands and fingers to create a cup shape. Rhythmically tap the body with cupped hands starting with the upper limbs and moving all the way down to the ankles. Cupping has many benefits, including increased blood flow and release of built-up fluids.

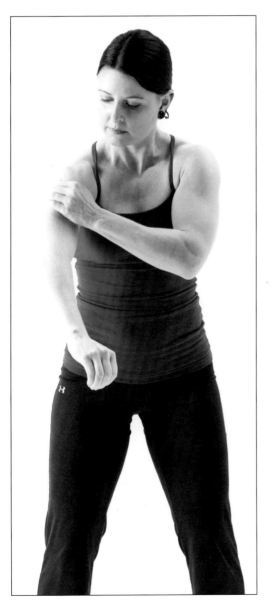
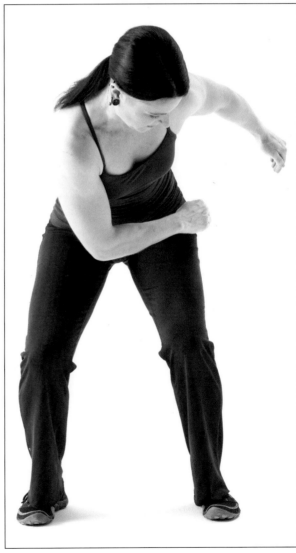

## Extreme Examples

I have used several extreme Neuro-Strike techniques to enhance my workout intensity. I have practiced controlled striking with rock filled canvas beating bags, Iron Palm bags, and a martial arts conditioning hammer. These techniques are extreme and are not recommended for beginners.

Choose one of the Neuro-Strike techniques that best works for you. Practice Neuro-Striking for a few minutes before your workout, and watch your intensity skyrocket.

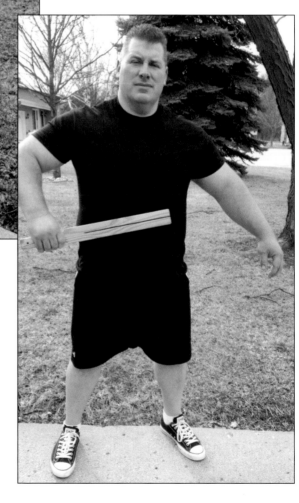

## The Neuro-Stomp

Our feet contain many nerve endings. These nerve endings are constantly sending information to the brain. By stimulating the nerves in the feet, the nervous system is more prepared to handle heavy weights. The technique is very simple. Stomp each foot into the ground one time before your workout and get ready to build smart muscle.

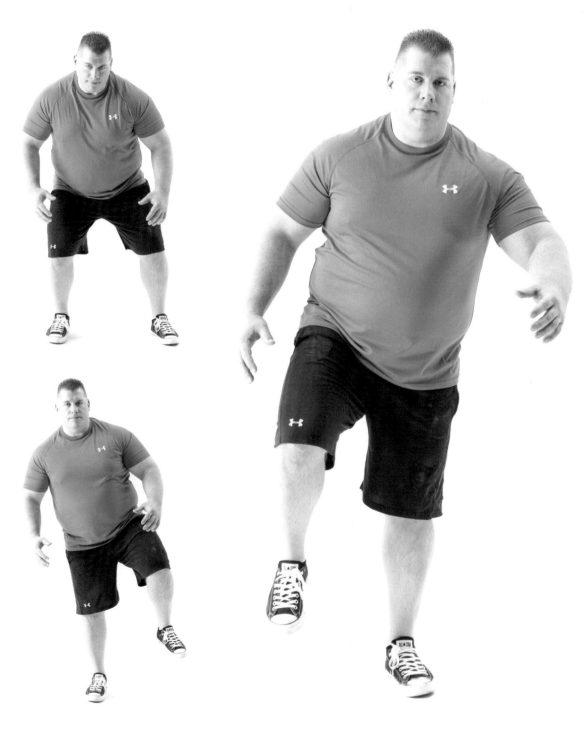

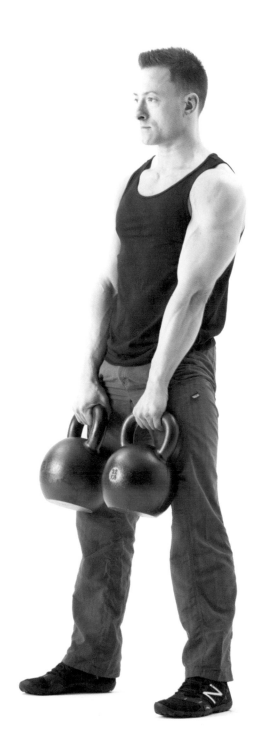

# Neuro-Recovery

ne of the key components in the Neuro-Mass program is recovery. Due to the extreme intensity of Neuro-Set training is essential to use recovery methods to continue building smart muscle. The following Neuro-Recovery techniques will enhance your recovery rate.

## Slow Abdominal Breathing

Start by standing with your feet shoulder width apart and relaxed knees. Slowly inhale through the nose and expand your abdomen. Pause for a moment, and slowly exhale. Repeat this breathing cycle for at least 10 times. Slow abdominal breathing creates a calming sensation, combats stress, improves sleep, and can activate the parasympathetic system. Practice this technique anytime you need to relax and recover.

## Far Infrared Sauna

Far infrared rays have many benefits for athletes. Far infrared saunas create radiant, penetrating heat that increases circulation. This brings about increased recovery to the muscles and joints as oxygen flow is enhanced. Other benefits include increased flexibility, detoxification, pain relief, and lower blood pressure. A far infrared sauna session is the perfect complement to a great Neuro-Set workout.

## Circulation Showers

This is a fantastic technique to speed your recovery. Stand in a hot shower with the heat set to a temperature that you can withstand. After 1 minute, switch the water to cold. Stand in the cold water for 1 minute before switching the temperature back to hot. Repeat this back and forth cycle or at least 6 minutes. Another benefit to circulation showers is that they increase the body's adaptability to stress.

### Binaural Beats and Isochronic Tones

This technology uses aural stimulus to create brainwave frequencies. The aural stimulus of binaural beats or isotonic tones can assist individuals in achieving certain brainwave states. Theta and Delta frequencies are ideal for relaxation and inducing sleep. There are many programs available utilizing this technology.

### Foam Rolling

Foam rolling is an excellent way to perform myofascial release techniques and increase recovery. Foam rollers use your own bodyweight to increase flexibility, circulation, and healing of muscles. Use this technique following a Neuro-Set workout to jumpstart your recovery.

# Neuro-Blitz Nutritional Timing

Neuro-Blitz nutritional timing will help maximize your gains in the Neuro-Mass program. We want to take advantage of the hormonal response to food and exercise. To accomplish this, timing is essential. The following are simple nutritional guidelines that can make a big difference in your quest for smart muscle.

### Natural Growth Hormone Response

The Neuro-Set training along with the proper timing of meals will create a natural release of growth hormone. The key is exercising on an empty stomach, or what we call a fasted state. Not everyone is able to do this, but those who are can take full advantage of this hormonal boost. My recommendation is to limit, not restrict carbohydrates in the meal leading up to your workout. The pre-workout meal should be 90 min. to 120 min. before the workout, and should be primarily protein. Make sure that you are properly hydrated. If you take a pre-workout energy supplement, make sure that it is carbohydrate free. Performing the intense exercises of the Neuro-Mass program in a fasted state will create a great surge of growth hormone.

## The Neuro-Blitz Shake

Immediately following the workout, you want to blitz the body with smart muscle building nutrients. The Neuro-Set training primes the body to receive nutrients in a maximal way. We also want to blunt the effects of cortisol, so it is essential to drink a Neuro-Blitz shake within a half-hour of the completion of your workout.

### The Neuro-Blitz Shake Ingredients and Supplements

Here are the ingredients of the Neuro-Blitz shake and supplements to take along with it.

### Neuro-Blitz shake:

- Protein – 30 to 40 g.
- Waxy maize starch or other carbohydrate source – 10 to 20 g
- Branched chain amino acids – 5 to 10 g
- L-glutamine – 5 g
- Powdered greens – 1 to 2 tablespoons

### Supplements

- Multivitamin
- Vitamin C – 1000 mg
- Vitamin D3 – 1000 to 2000 mg
- Fish oil – 1200 mg
- Probiotics

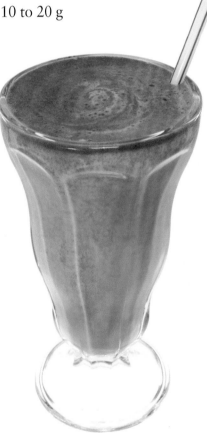

### The Evening Meal

In the evening we want to activate the parasympathetic system. This meal should include plenty of carbohydrates, protein, and healthy fats. It is also essential to include cruciferous vegetables as they will help hormonally.

This simple eating plan will deliver great gains.

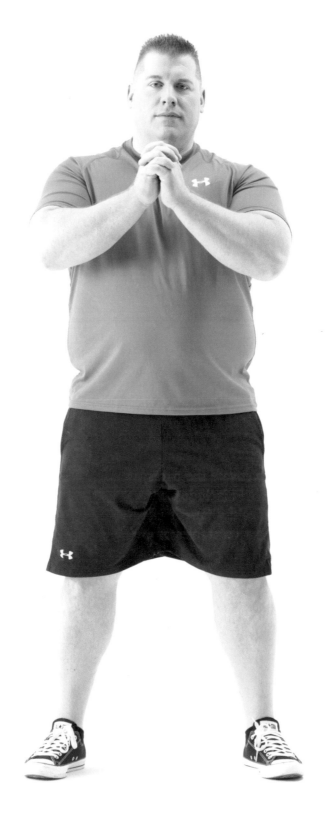

# Conclusion

*"Always bear in mind that your own resolution to succeed is more important than any one thing."*
*— Abraham Lincoln*

ow, you have the knowledge to build smart muscle. Go and succeed in your quest.

I'm looking forward to hearing about your success!

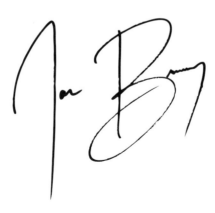

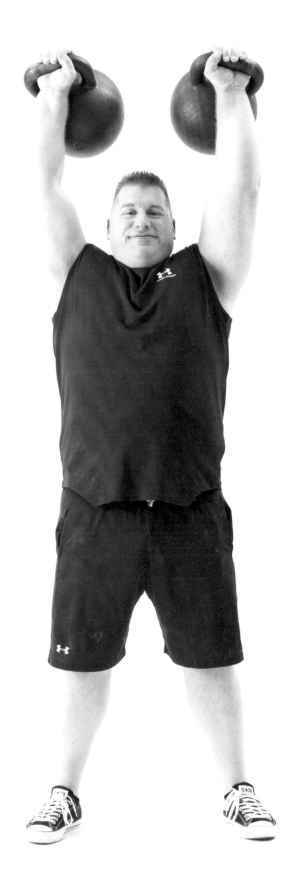

# About the Author

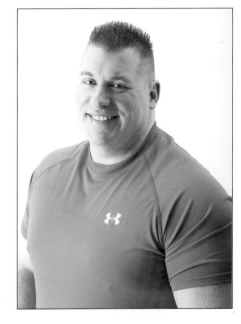

The exploits of World Record-holding strongman Jon Bruney have been immortalized in *Ripley's Believe it or Not* and shown nationwide on NBC's *The Today Show*. Thousands of people have personally experienced Jon's jaw-dropping "Pressing the Limits" motivational strength programs.

A true renaissance man in the realm of strength-development, Jon Bruney is a world-class trainer, coach, motivational speaker, strongman, author, and pastor. Jon's work with competitive athletes includes Olympians and NFL players. He is the author of *Foundations*, a training series featured in *MILO*, widely considered the world's most prestigious strength training journal. As co-owner of Submit Strength Equipment, Jon has been responsible for the design of numerous pieces of cutting-edge training equipment now in use around the world. Jon is a veteran of numerous trainer certification courses including Battling Ropes Level Two Coach and Controlled Fatigue Training.

Jon's passion is to help individuals reach their physical, mental, and spiritual potential. To learn more about Jon or to find information about speaking and training engagements, check out:
www.pressingthelimits.com
www.submitstrength.com

# Build Your Body To Be Ripped, Rugged and Spectacular—With Dragon Door's Best-of-Class, RKC Kettlebell

## The Ultimate "Handheld Gym"— Designed for A Lifetime of Hard, High-Performance Use...

**E**ven a man of average initial strength can immediately start using the 16kg/35lb kettlebell for two-handed swings and quickly gravitate to one-handed swings, followed by jerks, cleans and snatches. Within a few weeks you can expect to see spectacular gains in overall strength and conditioning—and for many—significant fat loss.

Dragon Door re-introduced kettlebells to the US with the uniquely designed 35lb cast iron kettlebell—and it has remained our most popular kettlebell. Why? Let Dragon Door's own satisfied customers tell the story:

### Excellent Quality

"Unlike other kettlebells I have used, Dragon Door is of far superior quality. You name it, Dragon Door has got it! Where other bells lack, Dragon Door kettlebells easily meet, if not exceed, what a bell is supposed to have in quality! Great balance, nice thick handle for grip strength, and a finish that won't destroy your hands when doing kettlebell exercises."
—Barry Adamson, Frederick, MD

### New Dragon Door Bells— Best Ever!

"Just received a new e-coat 16 yesterday. Perfect balance, perfect texturing, non-slip paint, and absolutely seamless."
—Daniel Fazzari, Carson City, NV

### Continually Impressed

"Dragon Door never fails to impress with their quality service and products. I bought the 16kg last month and since adding it to my kettlebell 'arsenal', I am seeing huge improvement from the heavier weight. I have larger hands for a woman so the handle on the 16kg fits my hands perfectly and it feels great…This is my fifth month using kettlebells and I cannot imagine NOT using them. They have changed my life." —Tracy Ann Mangold, Combined Locks, WI

### Dragon Door bells just feel better

"I purchased this 35lb bell for a friend, and as I was carrying it to him I was thinking of ways I could keep it for myself. Everything about this bell is superior to other brands. The finish is the perfect balance of smooth and rough. The handle is ample in both girth and width even for a 35 lb bell, and the shape/dimensions make overhead work so much more comfortable. There is a clear and noticeable difference between Dragon Door bells and others. Now I am looking to replace my cheap bells with Dragon Door's. On a related note, my friend is thrilled with his bell."—Raphael Sydnor, Woodberry Forest, VA

### Made for Heavy-Duty Use!

"These kettlebells are definitely made for heavy-duty use! They are heftier than they appear, and the centrifugal force generated while swinging single or two-handed requires correct form. I have read numerous online reviews of different companies who manufacture kettlebells, and it I have yet to read a negative review of the kettlebells sold by Dragon Door. I have both the 35 and 44 lbs KBs, and I expect to receive a 53 lbs KB from Dragon Door by next week. And as I gain in strength and proficiency I will likely order the 72 lbs KB. If you like to be challenged physically and enjoy pushing yourself, then buy a Russian Kettlebell and start swinging!"
—Mike Davis, Newman, CA

### Dragon Door Kettlebells: The Real Deal!

"The differences between Dragon Door's authentic Russian kettlebell and the inferior one which I had purchased earlier at a local big box sports store are astounding! The Dragon Door design and quality are clearly superior, and your kettlebell just 'feels right in my hand. There is absolutely no comparison (and yes, I returned the substandard hunk of iron to the big box store for a credit as soon as I received your kettlebell). I look forward to purchasing a heavier kettlebell from dragondoor.com as soon as I master the 16kg weight!"—Stephen Williams, Arlington, VA

**MONEY BACK GUARANTEE ONE YEAR**

## CALL NOW: 1-800-899-5111  OR VISIT: www.dragondoor.com

# Whatever Your Athletic Challenge, Dragon Door Has the Perfect Kettlebell Size to Meet Your Demand!

## Classic Russian Kettlebells—All Cast Iron/E-Coated

 **Russian Kettlebell 10 lbs.**
#P10N $41.75
*Call for shipping costs*

 **Russian Kettlebell 16kg (35 lbs.)**
#P10A $96.75
*Call for shipping costs*

 **Russian Kettlebell 32kg (70 lbs.)**
#P10C $153.94
*Call for shipping costs*

 **Russian Kettlebell 14 lbs.**
#P10P $54.95
*Call for shipping costs*

 **Russian Kettlebell 18kg (40 lbs.)**
#P10W $102.75
*Call for shipping costs*

 **Russian Kettlebell 36kg (79 lbs.)**
#P10Q $175.95
*Call for shipping costs*

 **Russian Kettlebell 18 lbs.**
#P10M $65.95
*Call for shipping costs*

 **Russian Kettlebell 20kg (44 lbs.)**
#P10H $107.75
*Call for shipping costs*

 **Russian Kettlebell 40kg (88 lbs.)**
#P10F $197.65
*Call for shipping costs*

 **Russian Kettlebell 10kg (22 lbs.)**
#P10T $71.45
*Call for shipping costs*

 **Russian Kettlebell 22kg (48 lbs.)**
#P10X $112.75
*Call for shipping costs*

 **Russian Kettlebell 44kg (97 lbs.)**
#P10R $241.95
*Call for shipping costs*

 **Russian Kettlebell 12kg (26 lbs.)**
#P10G $76.95
*Call for shipping costs*

 **Russian Kettlebell 24kg (53 lbs.)**
#P10B $118.75
*Call for shipping costs*

 **Russian Kettlebell 48kg (106 lbs.)**
#P10L $263.95
*Call for shipping costs*

 **Russian Kettlebell 14kg (31 lbs.)**
#P10U $87.95
*Call for shipping costs*

 **Russian Kettlebell 28kg (62 lbs.)**
#P10J $142.95
*Call for shipping costs*

**ALASKA/HAWAII KETTLEBELL ORDERING**
Dragon Door now ships to all 50 states, including Alaska and Hawaii, via UPS Ground. 32kg and above available for RUSH (2-day air) shipment only.

**CANADIAN KETTLEBELL ORDERING**
Dragon Door now accepts online, phone and mail orders for Kettlebells to Canada, using UPS Standard service. UPS Standard to Canada service is guaranteed, fully tracked ground delivery, available to every address in all of Canada's 10 provinces. Delivery time can vary between 3 to 10 business days.

**IMPORTANT** — International shipping quotes & orders do not include customs clearance, duties, taxes or other non-routine customs brokerage charges, which are the responsibility of the customer.

· KETTLEBELLS ARE SHIPPED VIA UPS GROUND SERVICE, UNLESS OTHERWISE REQUESTED.
· KETTLEBELLS RANGING IN SIZE FROM 10 LBS. TO 24 KG CAN BE SHIPPED TO P.O. BOXES OR MILITARY ADDDRESSES VIA THE U.S. POSTAL SERVICE, BUT WE REQUIRE PHYSICAL ADDDRESSES FOR UPS DELIVERIES FOR ALL SIZES 32KG AND HEAVIER.

# CALL NOW: 1-800-899-5111 OR VISIT: www.dragondoor.com

# Go Beyond Mere "Toughness"— When You Master The Art of Bar Athletics and Sculpt the Ultimate in Upper Body Physiques

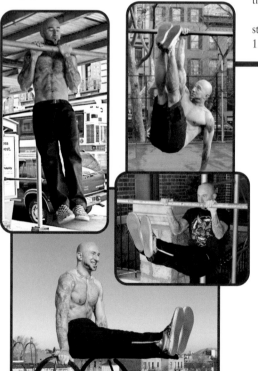

"*Raising the Bar* is very likely the most important book on strength and conditioning to be published in the last fifty years. If you only ever get your hands on one training manual in your life, make it this one. Buy it, read it, use it. This book has the power to transform you into the ultimate bar athlete."
—**Paul "Coach" Wade**, author of *Convict Conditioning*

**Raising the Bar**
*The Definitive Guide to Bar Calisthenics*
**By Al Kavadlo**    **#B63  $39.95**
224 pages, 330 Photos

**1** Beginner  **2** Mid-Level  **3** Advanced

**R**aising the Bar breaks down every type of exercise you can do with a pull-up bar. From the basic two arm hang, to the mighty muscle-up, all the way to the elusive one arm pull-up, "bar master" Al Kavadlo takes you step by expert step through everything you need to do to build the chiseled frame you've always wanted.

Whether you're a die-hard calisthenics enthusiast or just looking to get in the best shape of your life, *Raising the Bar* will meet all your expectations—and then some!

The message is clear: you can earn yourself a stunning upper body with just 3 basic moves and 1 super-simple, yet amazingly versatile tool.

And what's even better, this 3 + 1 formula for upper body magnificence hides enough variety to keep you challenged and surging to new heights for a lifetime of cool moves and ever-tougher progressions!

Cast in the "concrete jungle" of urban scaffolding and graffiti-laden, blasted walls—and sourced from iconic bar-athlete destinations like Tompkins Square Park, NYC—*Raising the Bar* rears up to grab you by the throat and hurl you into an inspiring new vision of what the human body can achieve. Embrace Al Kavadlo's vision, pick up the challenge, share the Quest, follow directions—and the Holy Grail of supreme upper body fitness is yours for the taking.

"With *Raising the Bar*, Al Kavadlo has put forth the perfect primal pull-up program. Al's progressions and demonstrations make even the most challenging exercises attainable. Anyone who is serious about pull-ups should read this book."—**Mark Sisson**, author of *The Primal Blueprint*.

**A Kick Ass Encyclopedia of Bodyweight Exercises**

"Al Kavadlo has put together a kick ass encyclopedia of the most powerful and most commonly used bodyweight exercises amongst the various groups of bodyweight masters. From the most simple form of each exercise progressing to the most challenging form of each exercise, Al covers it. As a Coach and bodyweight training addict I loved all the variations shown. This book is far beyond just pull ups and there are countless exercises for upper body and abs. Al covers what is probably EVERY exercise he knows of, uses and teaches others, breaking down proper techniques, regressions and progressions. This is HUGE for the trainers out there who do NOT know how to adapt bodyweight exercises to each individual's fitness level.

If you're a fan of bodyweight training, between this book and *Convict Conditioning* you can turn your body into a deadly weapon!!!" —**Zach Even-Esh**, Manasquan, NJ

"Al has put together the companion manual for all the crazy bar calisthenics videos that you find yourself watching over and over again—a much needed resource. Within this book is a huge volume of bar exercises that will keep your pullup workouts fresh for years, and give you some insane goals to shoot for."
—**Max Shank**, Senior RKC

"The only tool required to fully train bodyweight is a bar or something to hang on. I believe that this amazing book by Al Kavadlo, contains everything that is ever possible to do with a bar, from entry level to 'mutant' level. Thanks to the information contained in this book you will have material to practice and improve your skills for years"—**Fabio Zonin**, Senior RKC, Italian bodybuilding champion, Master Instructor FIF

# How Do YOU Stack Up Against These 6 Signs of a TRUE Physical Specimen?

## According to Paul Wade's *Convict Conditioning* you earn the right to call yourself a "true physical specimen" if you can perform the following:

✔ 1. AT LEAST one set of 5 one-arm pushups each side— with the ELITE goal of 100 sets each side

✔ 2. AT LEAST one set of 5 one-leg squats each side— with the ELITE goal of 2 sets of 50 each side

✔ 3. AT LEAST a single one-arm pullup each side— with the ELITE goal of 2 sets of 6 each side

✔ 4. AT LEAST one set of 5 hanging straight leg raises— with the ELITE goal of 2 sets of 30

✔ 5. AT LEAST one stand-to-stand bridge— with the ELITE goal of 2 sets of 30

✔ 6. AT LEAST a single one-arm handstand pushup on each side— with the ELITE goal of 1 set of 5

## Well, how DO you stack up?

C hances are that whatever athletic level you have achieved, there are some serious gaps in your OVERALL strength program. Gaps that stop you short of being able to claim status as a truly accomplished strength athlete.

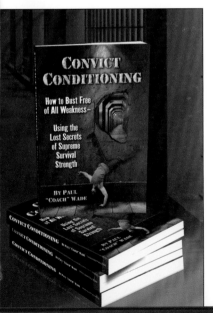

The good news is that—in *Convict Conditioning*—Paul Wade has laid out a brilliant 6-set system of 10 progressions which allows you to master these elite levels.

And you could be starting at almost any age and in almost in any condition...

Paul Wade has given you the keys—ALL the keys you'll ever need— that will open door, after door, after door for you in your quest for supreme physical excellence. Yes, it will be the hardest work you'll ever have to do. And yes, 97% of those who pick up *Convict Conditioning*, frankly, won't have the guts and the fortitude to make it. But if you make it even half-way through **Paul's Progressions**, you'll be stronger than almost anyone you encounter. Ever.

## Here's just a small taste of what you'll get with *Convict Conditioning:*

Can you meet these 5 benchmarks of the *truly powerful?*... Page 1

The nature and the art of real strength... Page 2

Why mastery of *progressive calisthenics* is the ultimate secret for building maximum raw strength... Page 2

A dozen one-arm handstand pushups without support— anyone? Anyone?... Page 3

How to rank in a powerlifting championship—*without ever training with weights*... Page 4

Calisthenics as a hardcore strength training technology... Page 9

Spartan "300" calisthenics at the Battle of Thermopylae... Page 10

How to cultivate the perfect body—the Greek and Roman way... Page 10

The difference between "old school" and "new school" calisthenics... Page 15

The role of prisons in preserving the older systems... Page 16

Strength training as a primary survival strategy... Page 16

The 6 basic benefits of bodyweight training... Pages 22—27

Why calisthenics are the *ultimate* in functional training... Page 23

The value of cultivating s*elf-movement*—rather than *object-movement*... Page 23

The *real* source of strength—it's not your *muscles*... Page 24

One crucial reason why a lot of convicts deliberately avoid weight-training... Page 24

How to progressively strengthen your joints over a lifetime—and even heal old joint injuries... Page 25

Why "authentic" exercises like pullups are so perfect for strength and power development... Page 25

Bodyweight training for quick physique perfection... Page 26

How to normalize and regulate your body fat levels—with bodyweight training only... Page 27

Why weight-training and the psychology of overeating go hand in hand... Page 27

The best approach for rapidly strengthening your whole body is this... Page 30

This is the most important and revolutionary feature of *Convict Conditioning*.... Page 33

A jealously-guarded system for going from puny to powerful— when your life may depend on the speed of your results... Page 33

The 6 "Ultimate" Master Steps—only a handful of athletes in the whole world can correctly perform them all. Can you?... Page 33

How to Forge Armor-Plated Pecs and Steel Triceps... Page 41

Why the pushup is the *ultimate* upper body exercise—and better than the bench press... Page 41

How to effectively bulletproof the vulnerable rotator cuff muscles... Page 42

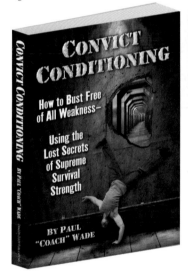

# Dragon Door Customer Acclaim for Paul Wade's *Convict Conditioning*

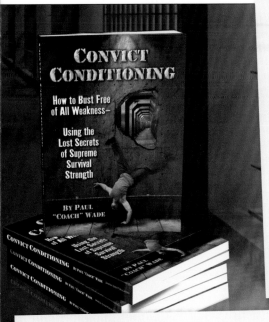

## A Strength Training Guide That Will Never Be Duplicated!

"I knew within the first chapter of reading this book that I was in for something special and unique. The last time I felt this same feeling was when reading *Power to the People!* To me this is the Body Weight equivalent to Pavel's masterpiece.

Books like this can never be duplicated. Paul Wade went through a unique set of circumstances of doing time in prison with an 'old time' master of calisthenics. Paul took these lessons from this 70 year old strong man and mastered them over a period of 20 years while 'doing time'. He then taught these methods to countless prisoners and honed his teaching to perfection.

I believe that extreme circumstances like this are what it takes to create a true masterpiece. I know that 'masterpiece' is a strong word, but this is as close as it gets. No other body weight book I have read (and I have a huge fitness library)...comes close to this as far as gaining incredible strength from body weight exercise.

Just like Power to the People, I am sure I will read this over and over again...mastering the principles that Paul Wade took 20 years to master.

Outstanding Book!"—*Rusty Moore - Fitness Black Book - Seattle, WA*

## A must for all martial artists

"As a dedicated martial artist for more than seven years, this book is exactly what I've been looking for.

For a while now I have trained with machines at my local gym to improve my muscle strength and power and get to the next level in my training. I always felt that the modern health club, technology based exercise jarred with my martial art though, which only required body movement.

Finally this book has come along. At last I can combine perfect body movement for martial skill with perfect body exercise for ultimate strength.

All fighting arts are based on body movement. This book is a complete textbook on how to max out your musclepower using only body movement, as different from dumbbells, machines or gadgets. For this reason it belongs on the bookshelf of every serious martial artist, male and female, young and old."—*Gino Cartier - Washington DC*

## I've packed all of my other training books away!

"I read CC in one go. I couldn't put it down. I have purchased a lot of bodyweight training books in the past, and have always been pretty disappointed. They all seem to just have pictures of different exercises, and no plan whatsoever on how to implement them and progress with them. But not with this one. The information in this book is AWESOME! I like to have a clear, logical plan of progression to follow, and that is what this book gives. I have put all of my other training books away. CC is the only system I am going to follow. This is now my favorite training book ever!"—*Lyndan - Australia*

## Brutal Elegance.

"I have been training and reading about training since I first joined the US Navy in the 1960s. I thought I'd seen everything the fitness world had to offer. Sometimes twice. But I was wrong. This book is utterly iconoclastic.

The author breaks down all conceivable body weight exercises into six basic movements, each designed to stimulate different vectors of the muscular system. These six are then elegantly and very intelligently broken into ten progressive techniques. You master one technique, and move on to the next.

The simplicity of this method belies a very powerful and complex training paradigm, reduced into an abstraction that obviously took many years of sweat and toil to develop.

Trust me. Nobody else worked this out. This approach is completely unique and fresh.

I have read virtually every calisthenics book printed in America over the last 40 years, and instruction like this can't be found anywhere, in any one of them. *Convict Conditioning* is head and shoulders above them all. In years to come, trainers and coaches will all be talking about 'progressions' and 'progressive calisthenics' and claim they've been doing it all along. But the truth is that Dragon Door bought it to you first. As with kettlebells, they were the trail blazers.

Who should purchase this volume? Everyone who craves fitness and strength should. Even if you don't plan to follow the routines, the book will make you think about your physical prowess, and will give even world class experts food for thought. At the very least if you find yourself on vacation or away on business without your barbells, this book will turn your hotel into a fully equipped gym.

I'd advise any athlete to obtain this work as soon as possible."—*Bill Oliver - Albany, NY, United States*

# www.dragondoor.com
# 1·800·899·5111

**Order Convict Conditioning online:**
www.dragondoor.com/B41

# More Dragon Door Customer Acclaim for *Convict Conditioning*

## Fascinating Reading and Real Strength

"Coach Wade's system is a real eye opener if you've been a lifetime iron junkie. Wanna find out how really strong (or weak) you are? Get this book and begin working through the 10 levels of the 6 power exercises. I was pleasantly surprised by my ability on a few of the exercises...but some are downright humbling. If I were on a desert island with only one book on strength and conditioning this would be it. (Could I staple Pavel's "Naked Warrior" to the back and count them as one???!) Thanks Dragon Door for this innovative new author."—*Jon Schultheis, RKC (2005) - Keansburg, NJ*

## Single best strength training book ever!

"I just turned 50 this year and I have tried a little bit of everything over the years: martial arts, swimming, soccer, cycling, free weights, weight machines, even yoga and Pilates. I started using *Convict Conditioning* right after it came out. I started from the beginning, like Coach Wade says, doing mostly step one or two for five out of the six exercises. I work out 3 to 5 times a week, usually for 30 to 45 minutes.

Long story short, my weight went up 14 pounds (I was not trying to gain weight) but my body fat percentage dropped two percent. That translates into approximately 19 pounds of lean muscle gained in two months! I've never gotten this kind of results with anything else I've ever done. Now I have pretty much stopped lifting weights for strength training. Instead, I lift once a week as a test to see how much stronger I'm getting without weight training. There are a lot of great strength training books in the world (most of them published by Dragon Door), but if I had to choose just one, this is the single best strength training book ever. BUY THIS BOOK. FOLLOW THE PLAN. GET AS STRONG AS YOU WANT. "—*Wayne - Decatur, GA*

## Best bodyweight training book so far!

"I'm a martial artist and I've been training for years with a combination of weights and bodyweight training and had good results from both (but had the usual injuries from weight training). I prefer the bodyweight stuff though as it trains me to use my whole body as a unit, much more than weights do, and I notice the difference on the mat and in the ring. Since reading this book I have given the weights a break and focused purely on the bodyweight exercise progressions as described by 'Coach' Wade and my strength had increased more than ever before. So far I've built up to 12 strict one-leg squats each leg and 5 uneven pull ups each arm.

I've never achieved this kind of strength before - and this stuff builds solid muscle mass as well. It's very intense training. I am so confident in and happy with the results I'm getting that I've decided to train for a fitness/bodybuilding comp just using his techniques, no weights, just to show for real what kind of a physique these exercises can build. In sum, I cannot recommend 'Coach' Wade's book highly enough - it is by far the best of its kind ever!"—*Mark Robinson - Australia, currently living in South Korea*

## A lifetime of lifting...and continued learning.

"I have been working out diligently since 1988 and played sports in high school and college before that. My stint the Army saw me doing calisthenics, running, conditioning courses, forced marches, etc. There are many levels of strength and fitness. I have been as big as 240 in my powerlifting/strongman days and as low as 185-190 while in the Army. I think I have tried everything under the sun: the high intensity of Arthur Jones and Dr. Ken, the Super Slow of El Darden, and the brutality of Dinosaur Training Brooks Kubic made famous.

This is one of the BEST books I've ever read on real strength training which also covers other just as important aspects of health; like staying injury free, feeling healthy and becoming flexible. It's an excellent book. He tells you the why and the how with his progressive plan. This book is a GOLD MINE and worth 100 times what I paid for it!"
—*Horst - Woburn, MA*

## This book sets the standard, ladies and gentlemen

"It's difficult to describe just how much this book means to me. I've been training hard since I was in the RAF nearly ten years ago, and to say this book is a breakthrough is an understatement. How often do you really read something so new, so fresh? This book contains a complete new system of calisthenics drawn from American prison training methods. When I say 'system' I mean it. It's complete (rank beginner to expert), it's comprehensive (all the exercises and photos are here), it's graded (progressions from exercise to exercise are smooth and pre-determined) and it's totally original. Whether you love or hate the author, you have to listen to him. And you will learn something. This book just makes SENSE. In twenty years people will still be buying it."—*Andy McMann - Ponty, Wales, GB*

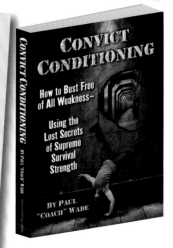

## Convict Conditioning
*How to Bust Free of All Weakness—Using the Lost Secrets of Supreme Survival Strength*
**By Paul "Coach" Wade**
**#B41 $39.95**
Paperback 8.5 x 11 320 pages
191 photos, charts and illustrations

**1** Beginner  **2** Mid-Level  **3** Advanced

# The Experts Give High Praise to
## *Convict Conditioning 2*

"Coach Paul Wade has outdone himself. His first book *Convict Conditioning* is to my mind THE BEST book ever written on bodyweight conditioning. Hands down. Now, with the sequel *Convict Conditioning 2*, Coach Wade takes us even deeper into the subtle nuances of training with the ultimate resistance tool: our bodies.

In plain English, but with an amazing understanding of anatomy, physiology, kinesiology and, go figure, psychology, Coach Wade explains very simply how to work the smaller but just as important areas of the body such as the hands and forearms, neck and calves and obliques in serious functional ways.

His minimalist approach to exercise belies the complexity of his system and the deep insight into exactly how the body works and the best way to get from A to Z in the shortest time possible.

I got the best advice on how to strengthen the hard-to-reach extensors of the hand right away from this exercise Master I have ever seen. It's so simple but so completely functional I can't believe no one else has thought of it yet. Just glad he figured it out for me.

Paul teaches us how to strengthen our bodies with the simplest of movements while at the same time balancing our structures in the same way: simple exercises that work the whole body.

And just as simply as he did with his first book. His novel approach to stretching and mobility training is brilliant and fresh as well as his take on recovery and healing from injury. Sprinkled throughout the entire book are too-many-to-count insights and advice from a man who has come to his knowledge the hard way and knows exactly of what he speaks.

This book is, as was his first, an amazing journey into the history of physical culture disguised as a book on calisthenics. But the thing that Coach Wade does better than any before him is his unbelievable progressions on EVERY EXERCISE and stretch! He breaks things down and tells us EXACTLY how to proceed to get to whatever level of strength and development we want. AND gives us the exact metrics we need to know when to go to the next level.

Adding in completely practical and immediately useful insights into nutrition and the mindset necessary to deal not only with training but with life, makes this book a classic that will stand the test of time.

Bravo Coach Wade, Bravo." —**Mark Reifkind, Master RKC,** author of *Mastering the HardStyle Kettlebell Swing*

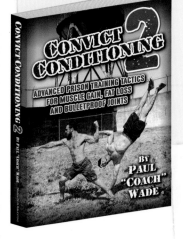

## Convict Conditioning 2
### *Advanced Prison Training Tactics for Muscle Gain, Fat Loss and Bulletproof Joints*
**By Paul "Coach" Wade**
**#B59   $39.95**
Paperback 8.5 x 11   354 pages
261 photos, charts and illustrations

**2** Mid-Level

**3** Advanced

"The overriding principle of *Convict Conditioning* 2 is 'little equipment-big rewards'. For the athlete in the throwing and fighting arts, the section on Lateral Chain Training, Capturing the Flag, is a unique and perhaps singular approach to training the obliques and the whole family of side muscles. This section stood out to me as ground breaking and well worth the time and energy by anyone to review and attempt to complete. Literally, this is a new approach to lateral chain training that is well beyond sidebends and suitcase deadlifts.

The author's review of passive stretching reflects the experience of many of us in the field. But, his solution might be the reason I am going to recommend this work for everyone: The Trifecta. This section covers what the author calls The Functional Triad and gives a series of simple progressions to three holds that promise to oil your joints. It's yoga for the strength athlete and supports the material one would find, for example, in Pavel's *Loaded Stretching*.

I didn't expect to like this book, but I come away from it practically insisting that everyone read it. It is a strongman book mixed with yoga mixed with street smarts. I wanted to hate it, but I love it."
—**Dan John,** author of *Don't Let Go* and co-author of *Easy Strength*

"I've been lifting weights for over 50 years and have trained in the martial arts since 1965. I've read voraciously on both subjects, and written dozens of magazine articles and many books on the subjects. This book and Wade's first, *Convict Conditioning,* are by far the most commonsense, information-packed, and result producing I've read. These books will truly change your life.

Paul Wade is a new and powerful voice in the strength and fitness arena, one that is commonsense, inspiring, and in your face. His approach to maximizing your body's potential is not the same old hackneyed material you find in every book and magazine piece that pictures steroid-bloated models screaming as they curl weights. Wade's stuff has been proven effective by hard men who don't tolerate fluff. It will work for you, too—guaranteed.

As an ex-cop, I've gone mano-y-mano with ex-cons that had clearly trained as Paul Wade suggests in his two *Convict Conditioning* books. While these guys didn't look like steroid-fueled bodybuilders (actually, there were a couple who did), all were incredibly lean, hard and powerful. Wade blows many commonly held beliefs about conditioning, strengthening, and eating out of the water and replaces them with result-producing information that won't cost you a dime." —**Loren W. Christensen,** author of *Fighting the Pain Resistant Attacker,* and many other titles

"*Convict Conditioning* is one of the most influential books I ever got my hands on. *Convict Conditioning 2* took my training and outlook on the power of bodyweight training to the 10th degree—from strengthening the smallest muscles in a maximal manner, all the way to using bodyweight training as a means of healing injuries that pile up from over 22 years of aggressive lifting.

I've used both *Convict Conditioning* and *Convict Conditioning 2* on myself and with my athletes. Without either of these books I can easily say that these boys would not be the BEASTS they are today. Without a doubt *Convict Conditioning 2* will blow you away and inspire and educate you to take bodyweight training to a whole NEW level."
—**Zach Even-Esh,** Underground Strength Coach

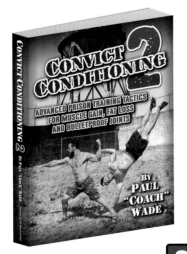

# TABLE OF CONTENTS

## Convict Conditioning 2

**2** Mid-Level

**3** Advanced

Advanced Prison Training Tactics for Muscle Gain, Fat Loss and Bulletproof Joints

**By Paul "Coach" Wade**
**#B59  $39.95**

Paperback 8.5 x 11  354 pages
261 photos, charts and illustrations

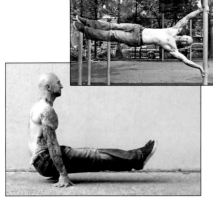

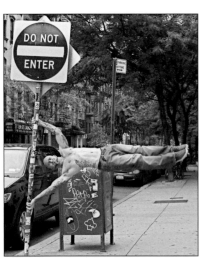

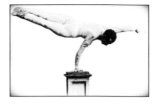
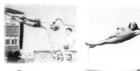

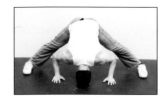
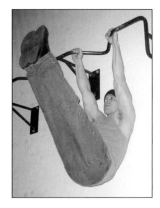
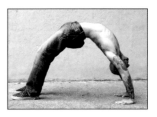
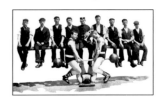

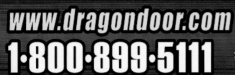

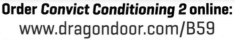

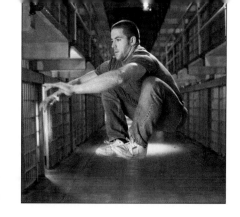

# GET DYNAMIC, CHISELLED, POWER-JACK LEGS AND DEVELOP EXPLOSIVE LOWER-BODY STRENGTH—WITH PAUL "COACH" WADE'S ULTIMATE BODYWEIGHT SQUAT COURSE

**P**aul Wade's *Convict Conditioning Ultimate Bodyweight Squat Course* explodes out of the cellblock to teach you in absolute detail how to progress from the ease of a simple shoulderstand squat—to the stunning "1-in-10,000" achievement of the prison-style one-leg squat. Ten progressive steps guide you to bodyweight squat mastery. Do it—and become a Bodyweight Squat Immortal.

This home-study course in ultimate survival strength comes replete with bonus material not available in **Paul Wade's** original *Convict Conditioning* book—and numerous key training tips that refine and expand on the original program.

A heavily and gorgeously-illustrated 80-plus-page manual gives you the entire film script to study at your leisure, with brilliant, precise photographs to remind you of the essential movements you absorbed in the DVD itself.

Paul Wade adds a bonus **Ten Commandments for Perfect Bodyweight Squats**—which is worth the price of admission alone. And there's the additional bonus of **5 major Variant drills** to add explosivity, fun and super strength to your core practice.

Whatever you are looking for from your bodyweight squats—be it supreme functional strength, monstrous muscle growth or explosive leg power—it's yours for the progressive taking with *Convict Conditioning, Volume 2: The Ultimate Bodyweight Squat Course.*

## WHY EVERY SELF-RESPECTING MAN WILL BE RELIGIOUS ABOUT HIS SQUATS...

Leg training is vital for every athlete. A well-trained, muscular upper body teetering around on skinny stick legs is a joke. Don't be that joke! The mighty squat is the answer to your prayers. Here's why:

- Squats train virtually every muscle in the lower body, from quads and glutes to hips, lower back and even hamstrings.

- Squat deep—as we'll teach you—and you will seriously increase your flexibility and ankle strength.

- All functional power is transmitted through the legs, so without strong, powerful legs you are *nothing*—that goes for running, jumping and combat sports as much as it does for lifting heavy stuff.

## ARE YOU FAILING TO BUILD MONSTROUS LEGS FROM SQUATS—BECAUSE OF THESE MISTAKES?

Most trainees learn how to squat on two legs, and then make the exercise harder by slapping a barbell across their back. In prison, this way of adding strength wasn't always available, so cell trainees developed ways of progressing using only bodyweight versus gravity. The best way to do this is to learn how to squat all the way down to the ground and back up on just one leg.

Not everybody who explores prison training will have the dedication and drive to achieve strength feats like the one-arm pullup, but the legs are much stronger than the arms. If you put

in the time and work hard, the one-leg squat will be within the reach of almost every athlete who pays their dues.

But the one-leg squat still requires very powerful muscles and tendons, so you don't want to jump into one-leg squatting right away. You need to build the joint strength and muscle to safely attempt this great exercise. Discover how to do that safely, using ten steps, ten progressively harder squat exercises.

## IN THE STRENGTH GAME, FOOLS RUSH IN WHERE ANGELS FEAR TO TREAD

The wise old Chinese man shouted to his rickshaw driver: "Slow down, young man, I'm in a hurry!" If ever a warning needed to be shouted to our nation of compulsive strength-addicts, this would be it. You see them everywhere: the halt, the lame, the jacked-up, the torn, the pain-ridden—the former glory-seekers who have been reduced to sad husks of their former selves

by rushing helter-skelter into heavy lifting without having first built a firm foundation.

Paul Wade reveals the ten key points of perfect squat form. The aspects of proper form apply to all your squats, and they'll not only unlock the muscle and power-building potential of each rep you do, but they'll also keep you as safe as you can be.

Bodyweight training is all about improving strength and health, not building up a list of injuries or aches and pains. They are so fundamental, we call them the Ten Commandments of good squat form.

Obey the Ten Commandments, follow the brilliantly laid out progressions religiously and you simply CANNOT fail to get stronger and stronger and stronger and stronger and stronger—surely, safely and for as long as you live…

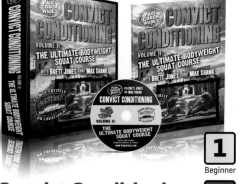

## Convict Conditioning
### Volume 2: The Ultimate Bodyweight Squat Course
**By Paul "Coach" Wade featuring Brett Jones and Max Shank**
#DV084 $69.95
DVD 56 minutes with full color Companion Manual, 88 pages

**1** Beginner

**2** Mid-Level

**3** Advanced

## COMPLEX MADE SIMPLE

Having read both *Convict Conditioning* and *Convict Conditioning 2*, the complementary DVD series is an excellent translation of the big six movement progressions into a simple to follow DVD. The demonstration of movement progression through the 10 levels is well described and easy to follow.

As a Physical Therapist it is a very useful way to teach safe progressions to patients/clients and other professionals. I have already used Volume I (the push up progression) to teach high school strength coaches how to safely progress athletes with pressing activity and look forward to using volume 2 with these same coaches. I think anyone who studies movement realizes very few athletes can properly squat with two legs, let alone one.

You will not find an easier way to teach the squat. Well done again Paul. Look forward to the rest of the series."
—Andrew Marchesi PT/MPT, FAFS, Scottsdale, AZ

## NAVY SEAL ON THE ROAD

"My whole team uses it. We can work out effectively anywhere and I mean anywhere!"
—Tyler Archer, Navy

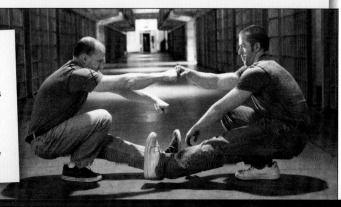

# GET A ROCK-HARD, BRUTISHLY POWERFUL UPPER FRAME AND ACHIEVE ELITE-LEVEL STRENGTH— WITH PAUL "COACH" WADE'S PRISON-STYLE PUSHUP PROGRAM

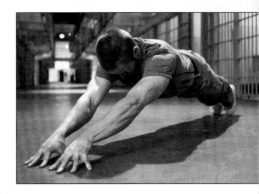

**P**aul Wade's *Convict Conditioning* system represents the ultimate distillation of hardcore prison bodyweight training's most powerful methods. What works was kept. What didn't, was slashed away. When your life is on the line, you're not going to mess with less than the absolute best. Many of these older, very potent solitary training systems have been on the verge of dying, as convicts begin to gain access to weights, and modern "bodybuilding thinking" floods into the prisons.

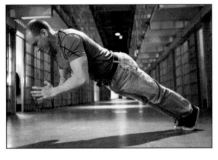

Thanks to Paul Wade, these ultimate strength survival secrets have been saved for posterity. And for you...

Filmed entirely—and so appropriately—on "The Rock", Wade's *Convict Conditioning Prison Pushup Series* explodes out of the cellblock to teach you in absolute detail how to progress from the ease of a simple wall pushup—to the stunning "1-in-10,000" achieve-ment of the prison-style one-arm pushup. Ten progressive steps guide you to pushup mastery. Do it—and become a Pushup God.

This home-study course in ultimate survival strength comes replete with bonus material not available in **Paul Wade's** original *Convict Conditioning* book—and numerous key training tips that refine and expand on the original program.

A heavily and gorgeously-illustrated 80-plus-page manual gives you the entire film script to study at your leisure, with brilliant, precise photographs to remind you of the essential movements you absorbed in the DVD itself.

Paul Wade adds a bonus **Ten Commandments for Perfect Pushups**—which is worth the price of admission alone. And there's the additional bonus of **5 major Variant drills** to add explosivity, fun and super-strength to your core practice.

Whatever you are looking for from your pushups—be it supreme functional strength, monstrous muscle growth or explosive upper-body power—it's yours for the progressive taking with *Convict Conditioning, Volume 1: The Prison Pushup Series.*

## AWESOME RESOURCE FOR COACHES & STRENGTH DEVOTEES

"I am using this manual and DVD not just for my own training, but for the training of my athletes. It shocks and amazes me how varsity high school athletes can NOT perform a solid push up.... not even 1! Getting them to perform a perfect push up requires regressions, progressions, dialing in the little cues that teach them to generate tension and proper body alignment, ALL of which carry over to other exercises.

This manual is an awesome resource for Coaches. It can & should be used to educate those you train as well as shared with your staff. For those who have a love for strength, you will respect all the details given for each and every push up progression and you will use them and apply them.

As a Strength devotee for over 2 decades, I've been through the grinder with free weights and injuries, push ups are something I KNOW I'll be doing for the rest of my life which is why I RESPECT this course so much!

The lay out of this manual and DVD are also BIG time impressive, the old school look and feel fires me up and makes me wanna attack these push ups!"
—Zach Even-Esh, Manasquan, NJ

## I RECOMMEND IT

"I fully expected to be disappointed with **Paul Wade's** *Convict Conditioning, Volume I: The Prison Pushup Series*. John Du Cane will tell you: I am not a fan of some of the stuff in these books. It's been said by others that this might be one of the most striking DVDs ever made. It's on location in Alcatraz and the graphics are pretty amazing. So, yes, stunning. This DVD from Wade is stunning and very cool.

The manual that supports the DVD is very helpful as much of the material is done too well in the DVD. Many of us need to take some time looking at the DVD then flipping the manual back and forth to 'get it.'

Once again, there are parts of this DVD and the series that rub me the wrong way. Having said that, I am frankly amazed at the insights of the product here. As a coach, I am better than when I popped the box open. I have a whole set of tools, and the progressions, that I can use tomorrow with my group. That to me is the testimony that people should hear from me: I watched it and I applied it instantly! This one 'gets it.' You can apply what you learn instantly and know where you are going from there. I highly recommend it."
—Dan John, Master RKC, Burlingame, CA

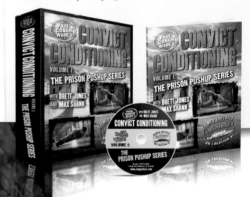

 **1** Beginner

 **2** Mid-Level

**3** Advanced

### Convict Conditioning
Volume 1: The Prison Pushup Series
**By Paul "Coach" Wade featuring Brett Jones and Max Shank**
**#DV083 $69.95**
DVD 59 minutes with full color Companion Manual, 88 pages

# DEMONIC ABS ARE A MAN'S BEST FRIEND—DISCOVER HOW TO SEIZE A SIX-PACK FROM HELL AND OWN THE WORLD... LEG RAISES

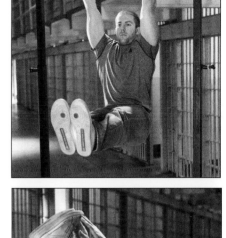

Paul Wade's *Convict Conditioning 3, Leg Raises: Six Pack from Hell* teaches you in absolute detail how to progress from the ease of a simple Knee Tuck—to the magnificent, "1-in-1,000" achievement of the Hanging Straight Leg Raise. Ten progressive steps guide you to inevitable mastery of this ultimate abs exercise. Do it, seize the knowledge—but beware—the Gods will be jealous!

This home-study course in ultimate survival strength comes replete with bonus material not available in **Paul Wade's** original *Convict Conditioning* book—and numerous key training tips that refine and expand on the original program.

Prowl through the heavily and gorgeously-illustrated 80-plus-page manual and devour the entire film script at your animal leisure. Digest the brilliant, precise photographs and reinforce the raw benefits you absorbed from the DVD.

Paul Wade adds a bonus **Ten Commandments for Perfect Bodyweight Squats**—which is worth the price of admission alone. And there's the additional bonus of **4 major Variant drills** to add explosivity, fun and super-strength to your core practice.

Whatever you are looking for when murdering your abs—be it a fist-breaking, rock-like shield of impenetrable muscle, an uglier-is-more-beautiful set of rippling abdominal ridges, or a monstrous injection of lifting power—it's yours for the progressive taking with *Convict Conditioning, Volume 3, Leg Raises: Six Pack from Hell*

## PRISON-STYLE MID-SECTION TRAINING—FOR AN ALL SHOW AND ALL GO PHYSIQUE

When convicts train their waists, they want real,

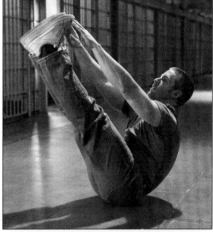

noticeable results—and by "results" we don't mean that they want cute, tight little defined abs. We mean that they want thick, strong, muscular midsections. They want *functionally* powerful abs and hips they can use for heavy lifting, kicking, and brawling. They want guts so strong from their training that it actually hurts an attacker to punch them in the belly. Prison abs aren't about all show, no go—a prison-built physique has to be all show and all go. Those guys don't just want six-packs—they want six-packs from Hell.

And, for the first time, we're going to show you how these guys get what they want. We're not going to be using sissy machines or easy isolation exercises—we're going straight for the old school secret weapon for gut training; progressive leg raises.

If you want a six-pack from Hell, the first thing you need to do is focus your efforts. If a weightlifter wanted a very thick, powerful chest in a hurry, he wouldn't spread his efforts out over a dozen exercises and perform them gently all day long. No—he'd pick just one exercise, probably the bench press, and just focus on getting stronger and stronger on that lift until he was monstrously strong. When he reached this level, and his pecs were thick slabs of meat, only then would he maybe begin sculpting them with minor exercises and higher reps.

It's no different if you want a mind-blowing midsection. Just pick one exercise that hits all the muscles in the midsection—the hip flexors, the abs, the intercostals, the obliques—then blast it.

And the one exercise we're going to discover is the best midsection exercise known to man, and the most popular amongst soldiers, warriors, martial artists and prison athletes since men started working out—the leg raise.

You'll discover ten different leg raise movements, each one a little harder than the last. You'll learn how to get the most out of each of these techniques, each of these ten steps, before moving up to the next step. By the time you get through all ten steps and you're working with the final Master Step of the leg raise series, you'll have a solid, athletic, stomach made of steel, as well as powerful hips and a ribcage armored with dense muscle. You'll have abs that would've made Bruce Lee take notice!

## THE TEN COMMANDMENTS YOU MUST OBEY TO EARN A REAL MONSTER OF AN ATHLETIC CORE

Paul Wade gives you ten key points, the "Ten Commandments" of leg raises, that will take your prison-style core training from just "okay" to absolutely phenomenal. We want the results to be so effective that they'll literally shock you. This kind of accelerated progress can be achieved, but if you want to achieve it you better listen carefully to these ten key pointers you'll discover with the DVD.

Bodyweight mastery is a lot like high-level martial arts. It's more about *principles* than individual techniques. Really study and absorb these principles, and you'll be on your way to a six-pack from Hell in no time.

The hanging straight leg raise, performed strictly and for reps, is the Gold Standard of abdominal strength techniques. Once you're at the level where you can throw out sets of twenty to thirty rock solid reps of this exercise, your abs will be thick and strong, but more importantly, they'll be functional—not just a pretty six-

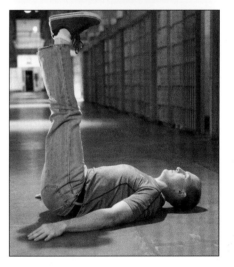

pack, but a real monster of an athletic core, which is capable of developing high levels of force.

Hanging will work your serratus and intercostals, making these muscles stand out like fingers, and your obliques and flank muscles will be tight and strong from holding your hips in place. Your lumbar spine will achieve a gymnastic level of flexibility, like fluid steel, and your chances of back pain will be greatly reduced.

The bottom line: If you want to be stronger and more athletic than the next guy, you need the edge that straight leg raises can give you.

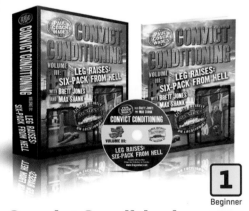

# ERECT TWIN PYTHONS OF COILED BEEF UP YOUR SPINE AND DEVELOP EXTREME, EXPLOSIVE RESILIENCE—WITH THE DYNAMIC POWER AND FLEXIBLE STRENGTH OF ADVANCED BRIDGING

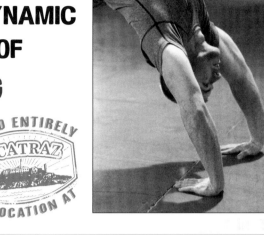

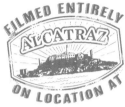

Paul Wade's *Convict Conditioning* system represents the ultimate distillation of hardcore prison body-weight training's most powerful methods. What works was kept. What didn't, was slashed away. When your life is on the line, you're not going to mess with less than the absolute best. Many of these older, very potent solitary training systems have been on the verge of dying, as convicts begin to gain access to weights, and modern "bodybuilding thinking" floods into the prisons. Thanks to Paul Wade, these ultimate strength survival secrets have been saved for posterity. And for you…

Filmed entirely—and so appropriately— on "The Rock", Wade's *Convict Conditioning Volume 4, Advanced Bridging: Forging an Iron Spine* explodes out of the cellblock to teach you in absolute detail how to progress from the relative ease of a Short Bridge—to the stunning, "1-in-1,000" achievement of the Stand-to-Stand Bridge. Ten progressive steps guide you to inevitable mastery of this ultimate exercise for an unbreakable back.

This home-study course in ultimate sur-

vival strength comes replete with bonus material not available in **Paul Wade's** original *Convict Conditioning* book—and numerous key training tips that refine and expand on the original program.

Prowl through the heavily and gorgeously-illustrated 80-plus-page manual and devour the entire film script at your animal leisure. Digest the brilliant, precise photographs and reinforce the raw benefits you absorbed from the DVD.

Paul Wade adds a bonus **Ten Commandments for Perfect Bridges**— which is worth the price of admission alone. And there's the additional bonus of **4 major Variant drills** to add explosivity, fun and super-strength to your core practice.

Whatever you are looking for from your pushups—be it supreme functional strength, monstrous muscle growth or explosive upper-body power—it's yours for the progressive taking with *Convict Conditioning Volume 4: Advanced Bridging: Forging an Iron Spine.*

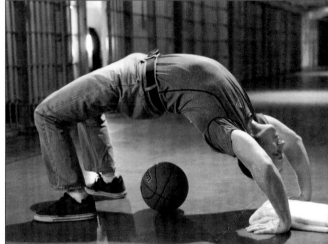

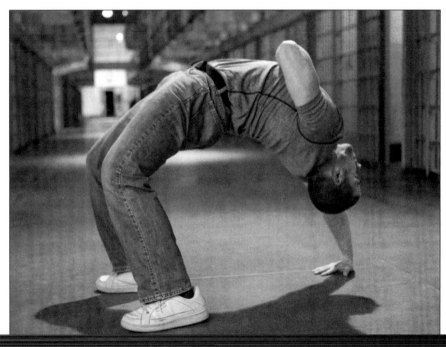

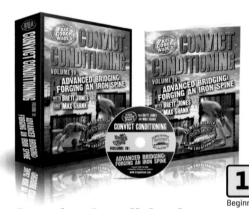

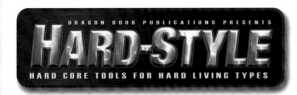

**DRAGON DOOR PUBLICATIONS PRESENTS**

# HARD-STYLE

### HARD CORE TOOLS FOR HARD LIVING TYPES

# 1·800·899·5111
## 24 HOURS A DAY
## FAX YOUR ORDER (866) 280-7619

# ORDERING INFORMATION

**Customer Service Questions?** Please call us between 9:00am– 11:00pm EST Monday to Friday at 1-800-899-5111. Local and foreign customers call 513-346-4160 for orders and customer service

**100% One-Year Risk-Free Guarantee.** If you are not completely satisfied with any product—we'll be happy to give you a prompt exchange, credit, or refund, as you wish. Simply return your purchase to us,

and please let us know why you were dissatisfied—it will help us to provide better products and services in the future. *Shipping and handling fees are non-refundable.*

**Telephone Orders** For faster service you may place your orders by calling Toll Free 24 hours a day, 7 days a week, 365 days per year. When you call, please have your credit card ready.

---

**Complete and mail with full payment to: Dragon Door Publications, 5 County Road B East, Suite 3, Little Canada, MN 55117**

## Please print clearly

### Sold To:                                    A

Name_____

Street_____

City_____

State _____ Zip _____

Day phone*_____
* Important for clarifying questions on orders

## Please print clearly

### SHIP TO: *(Street address for delivery)*    B

Name_____

Street_____

City_____

State _____ Zip _____

Email_____

### *Warning to foreign customers:*
**The Customs in your country may or may not tax or otherwise charge you an additional fee for goods you receive. Dragon Door Publications is charging you only for U.S. handling and international shipping. Dragon Door Publications is in no way responsible for any additional fees levied by Customs, the carrier or any other entity.**

| ITEM # | QTY. | ITEM DESCRIPTION | ITEM PRICE | A OR B | TOTAL |
|--------|------|------------------|------------|--------|-------|
|        |      |                  |            |        |       |
|        |      |                  |            |        |       |
|        |      |                  |            |        |       |
|        |      |                  |            |        |       |
|        |      |                  |            |        |       |
|        |      |                  |            |        |       |
|        |      |                  |            |        |       |
|        |      |                  |            |        |       |
|        |      |                  |            |        |       |
|        |      |                  |            |        |       |
|        |      |                  |            |        |       |

## HANDLING AND SHIPPING CHARGES · NO COD'S
**Total Amount of Order Add (Excludes kettlebells and kettlebell kits):**

| | | | |
|---|---|---|---|
| $00.00 to 29.99 | Add $6.00 | $100.00 to 129.99 | Add $14.00 |
| $30.00 to 49.99 | Add $7.00 | $130.00 to 169.99 | Add $16.00 |
| $50.00 to 69.99 | Add $8.00 | $170.00 to 199.99 | Add $18.00 |
| $70.00 to 99.99 | Add $11.00 | $200.00 to 299.99 | Add $20.00 |
| | | $300.00 and up | Add $24.00 |

*Canada and Mexico add $6.00 to US charges. All other countries, flat rate, double US Charges. See Kettlebell section for Kettlebell Shipping and handling charges.*

| | |
|---|---|
| *Total of Goods* | |
| *Shipping Charges* | |
| *Rush Charges* | |
| *Kettlebell Shipping Charges* | |
| *OH residents add 6.5% sales tax* | |
| *MN residents add 6.5% sales tax* | |
| *TOTAL ENCLOSED* | |

**METHOD OF PAYMENT** ❑ CHECK ❑ M.O. ❑ MASTERCARD ❑ VISA ❑ DISCOVER ❑ AMEX

Account No. *(Please indicate all the numbers on your credit card)*        EXPIRATION DATE

⬜⬜⬜⬜ ⬜⬜⬜⬜ ⬜⬜⬜⬜ ⬜⬜⬜⬜        ⬜⬜/⬜⬜

**Day Phone:** (___)_____

**Signature:** _____        **Date:** _____

**NOTE:** *We ship best method available for your delivery address. Foreign orders are sent by air. Credit card or International M.O. only. For* **RUSH** *processing of your order, add an additional $10.00 per address. Available on money order & charge card orders only.*

*Errors and omissions excepted. Prices subject to change without notice.*

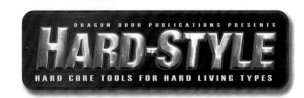

# ORDERING INFORMATION

## 1·800·899·5111
### 24 HOURS A DAY
### FAX YOUR ORDER (866) 280-7619

**Customer Service Questions?** Please call us between 9:00am– 11:00pm EST Monday to Friday at 1-800-899-5111. Local and foreign customers call 513-346-4160 for orders and customer service

**100% One-Year Risk-Free Guarantee.** If you are not completely satisfied with any product—we'll be happy to give you a prompt exchange, credit, or refund, as you wish. Simply return your purchase to us,

and please let us know why you were dissatisfied—it will help us to provide better products and services in the future. *Shipping and handling fees are non-refundable.*

**Telephone Orders** For faster service you may place your orders by calling Toll Free 24 hours a day, 7 days a week, 365 days per year. When you call, please have your credit card ready.

---

**Complete and mail with full payment to: Dragon Door Publications, 5 County Road B East, Suite 3, Little Canada, MN 55117**

## Please print clearly

### Sold To:                                     A

Name_____

Street_____

City_____

State _____ Zip _____

Day phone*_____
* Important for clarifying questions on orders

## Please print clearly

### SHIP TO: *(Street address for delivery)*   B

Name_____

Street_____

City_____

State _____ Zip _____

Email_____

### *Warning to foreign customers:*
**The Customs in your country may or may not tax or otherwise charge you an additional fee for goods you receive. Dragon Door Publications is charging you only for U.S. handling and international shipping. Dragon Door Publications is in no way responsible for any additional fees levied by Customs, the carrier or any other entity.**

| ITEM # | QTY. | ITEM DESCRIPTION | ITEM PRICE | A OR B | TOTAL |
|--------|------|------------------|------------|--------|-------|
|  |  |  |  |  |  |
|  |  |  |  |  |  |
|  |  |  |  |  |  |
|  |  |  |  |  |  |
|  |  |  |  |  |  |
|  |  |  |  |  |  |
|  |  |  |  |  |  |
|  |  |  |  |  |  |
|  |  |  |  |  |  |
|  |  |  |  |  |  |

## HANDLING AND SHIPPING CHARGES • NO COD'S
**Total Amount of Order Add (Excludes kettlebells and kettlebell kits):**

| | | | |
|---|---|---|---|
| $00.00 to 29.99 | Add $6.00 | $100.00 to 129.99 | Add $14.00 |
| $30.00 to 49.99 | Add $7.00 | $130.00 to 169.99 | Add $16.00 |
| $50.00 to 69.99 | Add $8.00 | $170.00 to 199.99 | Add $18.00 |
| $70.00 to 99.99 | Add $11.00 | $200.00 to 299.99 | Add $20.00 |
| | | $300.00 and up | Add $24.00 |

*Canada and Mexico add $6.00 to US charges. All other countries, flat rate, double US Charges. See Kettlebell section for Kettlebell Shipping and handling charges.*

| | |
|---|---|
| Total of Goods | |
| Shipping Charges | |
| Rush Charges | |
| Kettlebell Shipping Charges | |
| OH residents add 6.5% sales tax | |
| MN residents add 6.5% sales tax | |
| TOTAL ENCLOSED | |

**METHOD OF PAYMENT** ❐ CHECK ❐ M.O. ❐ MASTERCARD ❐ VISA ❐ DISCOVER ❐ AMEX

Account No. *(Please indicate all the numbers on your credit card)*          EXPIRATION DATE

☐☐☐☐ ☐☐☐☐ ☐☐☐☐ ☐☐☐☐          ☐☐/☐☐

**Day Phone:** (____)_____

**Signature:** _____     **Date:** _____

**NOTE:** *We ship best method available for your delivery address. Foreign orders are sent by air. Credit card or International M.O. only. For **RUSH** processing of your order, add an additional $10.00 per address. Available on money order & charge card orders only.*

*Errors and omissions excepted. Prices subject to change without notice.*

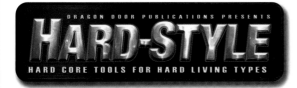

# ORDERING INFORMATION

## 1·800·899·5111
### 24 HOURS A DAY
### FAX YOUR ORDER (866) 280-7619

**Customer Service Questions?** Please call us between 9:00am– 11:00pm EST Monday to Friday at 1-800-899-5111. Local and foreign customers call 513-346-4160 for orders and customer service

**100% One-Year Risk-Free Guarantee.** If you are not completely satisfied with any product—we'll be happy to give you a prompt exchange, credit, or refund, as you wish. Simply return your purchase to us,

and please let us know why you were dissatisfied—it will help us to provide better products and services in the future. *Shipping and handling fees are non-refundable.*

**Telephone Orders** For faster service you may place your orders by calling Toll Free 24 hours a day, 7 days a week, 365 days per year. When you call, please have your credit card ready.

---

**Complete and mail with full payment to: Dragon Door Publications, 5 County Road B East, Suite 3, Little Canada, MN 55117**

### Please print clearly

**Sold To:**                                          **A**

Name_____

Street_____

City_____

State _____ Zip _____

Day phone*_____
* Important for clarifying questions on orders

### Please print clearly

**SHIP TO:** *(Street address for delivery)*     **B**

Name_____

Street_____

City_____

State _____ Zip _____

Email_____

**Warning to foreign customers:**
The Customs in your country may or may not tax or otherwise charge you an additional fee for goods you receive. Dragon Door Publications is charging you only for U.S. handling and international shipping. Dragon Door Publications is in no way responsible for any additional fees levied by Customs, the carrier or any other entity.

| ITEM # | QTY. | ITEM DESCRIPTION | ITEM PRICE | A OR B | TOTAL |
|--------|------|------------------|------------|--------|-------|
|        |      |                  |            |        |       |
|        |      |                  |            |        |       |
|        |      |                  |            |        |       |
|        |      |                  |            |        |       |
|        |      |                  |            |        |       |
|        |      |                  |            |        |       |
|        |      |                  |            |        |       |
|        |      |                  |            |        |       |
|        |      |                  |            |        |       |
|        |      |                  |            |        |       |
|        |      |                  |            |        |       |
|        |      |                  |            |        |       |

### HANDLING AND SHIPPING CHARGES • NO COD'S
**Total Amount of Order Add (Excludes kettlebells and kettlebell kits):**

| | | | |
|---|---|---|---|
| $00.00 to 29.99 | Add $6.00 | $100.00 to 129.99 | Add $14.00 |
| $30.00 to 49.99 | Add $7.00 | $130.00 to 169.99 | Add $16.00 |
| $50.00 to 69.99 | Add $8.00 | $170.00 to 199.99 | Add $18.00 |
| $70.00 to 99.99 | Add $11.00 | $200.00 to 299.99 | Add $20.00 |
| | | $300.00 and up | Add $24.00 |

*Canada and Mexico add $6.00 to US charges. All other countries, flat rate, double US Charges. See Kettlebell section for Kettlebell Shipping and handling charges.*

| |
|---|
| Total of Goods |
| Shipping Charges |
| Rush Charges |
| Kettlebell Shipping Charges |
| OH residents add 6.5% sales tax |
| MN residents add 6.5% sales tax |
| TOTAL ENCLOSED |

**METHOD OF PAYMENT** ❑ CHECK ❑ M.O. ❑ MASTERCARD ❑ VISA ❑ DISCOVER ❑ AMEX

Account No. *(Please indicate all the numbers on your credit card)*     EXPIRATION DATE

▢▢▢▢ ▢▢▢▢ ▢▢▢▢ ▢▢▢▢          ▢▢/▢▢

**Day Phone:** (___)_____

**Signature:** _____     **Date:** _____

---

**NOTE:** *We ship best method available for your delivery address. Foreign orders are sent by air. Credit card or International M.O. only. For* **RUSH** *processing of your order, add an additional $10.00 per address. Available on money order & charge card orders only.*

*Errors and omissions excepted. Prices subject to change without notice.*